AN INTRODUCTION TO
PHARMACOKINETICS

AN INTRODUCTION TO
PHARMACOKINETICS

BRUCE CLARK
BSc, PhD
Head of Toxicology
Fisons plc Pharmaceutical Division

DENNIS A. SMITH
BSc, MSc, PhD
Manager
Department of Drug Metabolism
Central Research
Pfizer Ltd

REVISED
SECOND EDITION

OXFORD

Blackwell Scientific Publications
LONDON EDINBURGH BOSTON
MELBOURNE PARIS BERLIN VIENNA

© 1981, 1986 by
Blackwell Scientific Publications
Editorial Offices:
Osney Mead, Oxford OX2 0EL
25 John Street, London WC1N 2BL
23 Ainslie Place, Edinburgh EH3 6AJ
238 Main Street, Cambridge
    Massachusetts 02142, USA
54 University Street, Carlton
    Victoria 3053, Australia

Other Editorial Offices:
Librairie Arnette SA
1, rue de Lille
75007 Paris
France

Blackwell Wissenschafts-Verlag
    GmbH
Düsseldorfer Str. 38
D-10707 Berlin
Germany

Blackwell MZV
Feldgasse 13
A-1238 Wien
Austria

First published 1981
Reprinted 1984
Second edition 1986
Reprinted 1990
Revised and reprinted 1993

Set by Setrite Typesetters, Hong Kong
Printed and bound in Great Britain at
the Alden Press, Oxford

DISTRIBUTORS

    Marston Book Services Ltd
    PO Box 87
    Oxford OX2 0DT
    (*Orders*: Tel: 0865 791155
             Fax: 0865 791927
             Telex: 837515)

USA
    Blackwell Scientific Publications,
        Inc.
    238 Main Street
    Cambridge, MA 02142
    (*Orders*: Tel: 800 759-6102
                 617 876-7000)

Canada
    Times Mirror Professional
        Publishing, Ltd
    130 Flaska Drive
    Markham, Ontario L6G 1B8
    (*Orders*: Tel: 800 268-4178
                 416 470-6739)

Australia
    Blackwell Scientific Publications
        Pty Ltd
    54 University Street
    Carlton, Victoria 3053
    (*Orders*: Tel: 03 347-5552)

A catalogue record for this title
is available from the British Library

ISBN 0-632-01559-4

Contents

Contents

Preface to revised second edition

It is now seven years since the second edition appeared and the explosion in pharmacokinetic methods and information has continued apace. Population kinetics and physiological modelling are just two particular areas of expansion. Despite all of this activity we are told that our simple basic text is still required. The principles outlined here have not changed and for this reason only minor changes and additions have been made in this edition. A few useful equations have been added. Our hope is that this volume will still continue to serve the purpose for which it was originally conceived.

B.C.
D.A.S.

Preface to first edition

This book was prompted when one of us had to give a series of lectures to medical students on the subject of pharmacokinetics. These lectures needed to start with the very basics of the subject. However, no simple introduction appeared to have been published to help either lecturer or student! Convinced that the essentials of pharmacokinetics could be understood without a profound knowledge of mathematics, we wrote the following text. Please remember that this is a simple introduction to what can be a very complex, although interesting, subject. Nevertheless, we believe that the simple basic concepts presented here will attract you as they have captivated us. We do not claim to be experts in pharmacokinetics but we do find ourselves using the concepts in this book almost daily in our work.

The text will be of use to students of pharmacy, pharmacology, human or veterinary medicine, toxicology and drug metabolism. It will also be useful background reading for others involved in the development and use of drugs. Sixth-form students of biology should not find the text too difficult and may find it of interest.

The text is presented in a special format since the mathematical treatment is restricted as far as possible to self-contained boxes. We suggest that you ignore these boxes on the first reading of the text. A second reading should, however, include the mathematical treatment. The material in the boxes can also be read and understood independently. Since this is an introductory text, some of the more complex concepts and mathematics are not included.

You will find it of great benefit to work through the examples given at the end of the book since these illustrate the main concepts discussed in the text.

B.C.
D.A.S.

List of common symbols

α, β	hybrid rate constants
AUC	area under curve
$\mathrm{AUC}_{0-\infty}$	area under the plasma (or blood)-concentration-versus-time curve from time zero to time infinity
$\mathrm{AUC}_{\mathrm{oral}}$ ⎫ $\mathrm{AUC}_{\mathrm{i.v.}}$ ⎭	area under the plasma (or blood)-concentration-versus-time curve for an oral dose and an i.v. dose of a drug, respectively
C_{p}	plasma concentration
$\bar{C}_{\mathrm{ss}}$	average steady-state plasma concentration
C_{ss}	steady-state plasma concentration
Cl	clearance
Cl_{B}	blood clearance
Cl_{P}	plasma clearance
D	drug
D_0	initial amount of drug
D_{u}	cumulative amount of unchanged drug excreted in urine
E	extraction (ratio or fraction)
F	fraction of an extravascular dose of drug which is absorbed
k_{ab}	absorption rate constant
k_{el}	elimination rate constant
k_{12}, k_{21}	rate constants for transfer of drug between compartments 1 and 2 in a two-compartment system
K_m	concentration at which half maximal rate occurs
Q_{B}	blood flow
t	time
$T_{1/2}$	half-life (half-time)
$T_{(1/2)\beta}$	biological half-life (terminal half-life in a multi-compartment system)
V_{C}	volume of central compartment
V_{D}	volume of distribution
V_{max}	maximal rate of drug elimination

Introduction

The *pharmacokineticist* seeks to understand how drugs act and behave, and to predict what they will do in new situations. The medical sciences owe much to the development of this relatively young discipline, *pharmacokinetics*.

Pharmacokineticists use words, symbols and mathematical equations to express and predict drug behaviour.

Words *describe what happens*. The concepts of pharmacokinetics can be explained in words. A profound understanding of mathematics is not necessary to grasp these principles.

Symbols *are used with defined meanings*. There is considerable confusion about the symbols used in publications on pharmacokinetics and for this reason the symbols used here are defined wherever necessary.

Mathematical equations *which are used here are functions* and show the relationships between one variable and another. The symbols and mathematics which form the language of pharmacokinetics are contained in boxes within the text of this book.

The subject of *kinetics* is concerned with the relationships between the motions of bodies and the forces acting upon them. Pharmacokinetics is therefore the science of the relationships between the movement of a drug through the body and the processes affecting it (i.e. the forces acting upon it). It is a discipline which describes the *time*-course of the movement of a drug into, around and out of the body.

Into the body. Most drugs need to be transported to their site of action by the blood. For the drug to be present in the blood following extravascular administration it needs to be *absorbed*. Absorption must therefore have taken place before a drug appears in the circulation after administration at an extravascular site. Drugs administered intramuscularly,

1

intraperitoneally, topically, orally, or *per rectum* need to be absorbed in order to appear in the circulation. Drugs administered intravenously and intra-arterially do not.

Around the body. Since the target organ or site is not usually the blood, the drug, once it is present in the circulation, must penetrate tissues in order to act. Drugs are not usually specific for a particular tissue and therefore will reach a number of tissues and organs. The drug can be said to be undergoing *distribution* when it is present in the blood and is penetrating organs and tissues.

Out of the body. *Elimination* is the removal of drug from the body and may be by renal and biliary excretion of the unchanged drug molecule or by metabolism. Two organs particularly important for eliminating drugs are the liver and the kidneys. With a few types of drugs other routes of elimination may assume importance, for example, in the case of volatile anaesthetics eliminated via the lungs.

Into

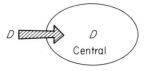

The drug (D) (◧▨) is absorbed into the central compartment from its site of administration.

(The central compartment is often equated with the blood but, in fact, it includes all those tissues and organs with which the drug is in rapid equilibrium.)

Around

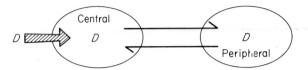

D distributes to peripheral compartment(s) in a reversible manner (⇌).

(The peripheral compartments are often equated with the tissues but, in pharmacokinetic terms, could include any areas in the body with which the drug equilibrates relatively slowly.)

Out

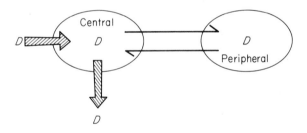

D is removed irreversibly (⇩) from the central compartment, that is, it is excreted or metabolized.

N.B. The above symbols represent a simple two-compartment model for the absorption, distribution and elimination of drugs. We will return to the concept of compartments later. In the mathematical treatment of most of the problems which follow we will use a simple one-compartment model, i.e.

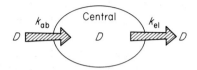

Where k_{ab} and k_{el} are constants which characterize the rate of movement of D.

In this model, all the tissues and organs to which D penetrates, behave as though they were in ready equilibrium with the blood.

 ## Rapid (bolus) intravenous injection

To study the mathematical equations which describe the above processes (movements *into*, *around* and *out* of the body) we must start with the simplest example. If we give someone a rapid intravenous injection (termed a bolus) of a drug, we introduce the drug directly into the blood and therefore we are, in effect, studying only the distribution and elimination. If the drug we have administered is very rapidly distributed, we have simplified the system even further so that we are studying only elimination. We can sample the blood, or more usually the plasma, for signs of the drug at various times. It is more usual to consider plasma concentrations of drug rather than blood concentrations since most assay methods are designed for plasma. In this book we will refer to plasma; however, the same terms can equally well apply to blood. The pharmacokinetic values calculated from plasma are not necessarily the same as those calculated from whole blood.

If we plot the results of our plasma concentration determinations against time, we will usually find that the concentration declines rapidly at first and then more and more slowly. If the method of analysis is sensitive enough, the rate of decline would eventually appear almost to stop. In practical terms, however, this represents such a minute quantity of the drug that it does not usually matter.

A relationship like this shows that the *rate* of removal of drug from the plasma changes continuously (in this case it decreases). In other words, the curve looks like an *exponential* decline and the rate of removal of the drug from the plasma is proportional to the amount present at a given time. This can be likened to the drug exerting a kind of 'pressure' to drive itself out: as the concentration of drug drops, so the 'pressure' decreases. Another way of describing this process is to say that a constant fraction of the drug present at any time is eliminated in unit time. This may be expressed as k_{el}, the elimination rate constant.

At first sight it is not easy to see why the removal of a drug from the plasma should take this form. In order to understand it, we must consider briefly the processes which contribute to the decline of drug in plasma. These are:

1 uptake by the liver and subsequent elimination in the bile,
2 elimination in the urine by glomerular filtration,
3 elimination in the urine by tubular secretion,
4 metabolism.

You may recognize that each of these processes is essentially one way (i.e. not reversible). Thus, drug is removed from the plasma and is not replaced. Furthermore, the rates at which these processes occur are proportional to the drug concentration driving them. Therefore, elimination from the plasma appears to be exponential. Uptake into the tissues has not been included with the routes of removal because this is normally a reversible process.

Volume of distribution

Consider the plasma concentration–time curve shown in Figure 1. The solid line represents the line drawn through a series of plasma concentration determinations.

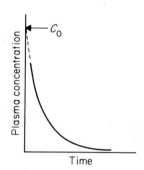

Figure 1

Extrapolation of the curve back to zero time would give an apparent value for the plasma concentration at zero time (C_0). It is evident that the total amount of drug in the body at zero time is given by this concentration multiplied by the volume in which the drug is distributed, assuming even distribution. This is the *volume of distribution*. The total amount of drug in the body at zero time in the case of a rapid intravenous dose is equal to the dose injected. Therefore, we can easily calculate this volume of distribution.

In practice, the extrapolation back to zero time is carried out much more conveniently using a $\log_{10}$ plasma concentration versus time curve as outlined on page 9.

It should be appreciated that this volume of distribution is an *apparent volume*, i.e. it does not necessarily reflect a literal volume of fluid in which the drug is dissolved. It includes, for example, tissues in which the drug, although in equilibrium with plasma, may be more highly concentrated than in the plasma. This explains why the reported volume of distribution often exceeds the total volume of the body.

Nevertheless, the volume of distribution of a drug often yields interesting information and it is related to several other parameters such as clearance.

A small volume of distribution (e.g. less than 5 litres in man) implies that the drug is largely retained within the vascular compartment. Distribution within the extracellular fluid would yield a volume of distribution of approximately 15 litres. Large volumes of distribution imply distribution throughout the total body water or concentration in certain tissues.

Rapid (bolus) intravenous injection

We usually find a decline in plasma concentration with time of the following form:

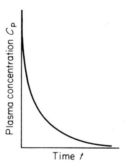

The mathematical relationship which appears to describe the above relationship fairly closely is of the general form:

$$X = X_0\, e^{-ky}$$

i.e. X at any given value of y is an exponential function of the starting value X_0 at $y = 0$.

It is a simple step to convert this equation for application to drugs:

$$D = D_0 \, e^{-k_{el}t}$$

where: D is the amount of drug in the body at time t;

D_0 is the initial amount of drug;

k_{el} is a constant which describes the rate of removal (elimination) of drug from the body (*the elimination rate constant*).

Thus, the rate of elimination of the drug varies continuously depending upon its concentration at any given time, i.e.

$$\frac{dD}{dt} \propto D$$

and therefore

$$\frac{dD}{dt} = -k_{el} \, D$$

The negative sign indicates that D decreases with time. This can be integrated to give:

$$D = D_0 \, e^{-k_{el}t}$$

Usually, a plasma, serum, or whole blood concentration of the drug is measured, whereas the above equation describes the total amount of drug in the body. Therefore, we need to introduce the concept of volume of distribution (V_D) to account for this.

If C_{P_t} = concentration in plasma at time t, then the total amount of drug in the body at time t is given by:

$$D = C_{P_t} \, V_D$$

where V_D is the *apparent* volume of distribution or for any value of time t

$$C_P = \frac{D_0}{V_D} e^{-k_{el}t}$$

or

$$C_P = C_0 \, e^{-k_{el}t}$$

C_0 is the theoretical initial plasma concentration at time t_0 after a bolus i.v. dose.

Log$_{10}$ plasma concentration versus time

Because the decline in plasma concentration behaves exponentially, it is usual to plot the results semi-logarithmically to obtain a straight line (Figure 2). The use of semi-logarithmic paper allows the plasma concentration to be plotted directly without using log$_{10}$ tables.

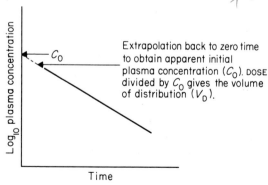

Extrapolation back to zero time to obtain apparent initial plasma concentration (C_0). DOSE divided by C_0 gives the volume of distribution (V_D).

Figure 2

By obtaining a linear plot we are able to extrapolate easily the straight line back to obtain the concentration of drug in plasma at time zero. This theoretical concentration is not measurable by sampling since mixing of the drug is not instantaneous. We are also governed in the obtainment of samples by ethical and practical constraints. Drugs are

Log$_{10}$ plasma concentration versus time

$$C_P = C_0 \, e^{-k_{el}t}$$

can be written

$$\ln C_P = \ln C_0 - k_{el}t$$

or

$$\log_{10} C_P = \log_{10} C_0 - \frac{k_{el}t}{2\cdot303}$$

Therefore, a plot of $\log_{10} C_P$ against time is linear with a slope of:

$$\frac{-k_{el}}{2\cdot303}$$

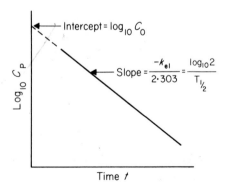

and intercept when $t = 0$ is given by:

$$\log_{10} C_0$$

When using semilogarithmic paper the slope is calculated by using the half-life.

not administered to patients solely for the purpose of carrying out pharmacokinetics.

The half-time (half-life) or $T_{1/2}$

The half-time ($T_{1/2}$) is the time taken for the concentration of drug in the blood or plasma to decline to half of its original value.

If the $\log_{10} C_P$ versus time plot is linear (Figure 3), then $T_{1/2}$ will be the same over the entire time period.

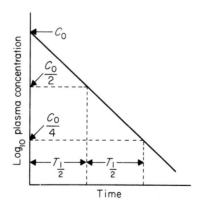

Figure 3

The elimination rate constant (k_{el}) is a constant which is more useful to the pharmacokineticist and it can be obtained by simple calculation from $T_{1/2}$. It is a proportionality constant, and may be defined as the fraction of drug present at any time which would be eliminated in unit time. For example, if k_{el} is $0{\cdot}1\,min^{-1}$, 10 per cent of the drug present at any instant in time would be eliminated in one minute. Note, however, that due to elimination the instantaneous concentration of drug present is continuously declining. Therefore, although the fraction eliminated remains constant, the actual rate of elimination declines with time.

The half-time (half-life) or $T_{1/2}$

When the concentration of drug in plasma or blood declines to half of its original value we have the relationship:

$$\frac{C_P}{C_0} = 0{\cdot}5$$

or, more generally, in the case of a linear $\log_{10} C_P$ versus t plot:

$$\frac{C_{P_t}}{C_{(t - T_{1/2})}} = 0{\cdot}5$$

where C_{P_t} is the concentration at time t and $C_{(t - T_{1/2})}$ is the concentration at a time $T_{1/2}$ earlier than t.

Since $\ln C_P = \ln C_0 - k_{el}\, t$

i.e. $\ln\left(\dfrac{C_P}{C_0}\right) = -k_{el}\, t$

and $\dfrac{C_P}{C_0} = 0{\cdot}5$ when $t = T_{1/2}$

then $\ln 0{\cdot}5 = -k_{el}\, T_{1/2}$

since $\ln 0{\cdot}5 = 0{\cdot}693$

$$T_{1/2} = \frac{0\cdot693}{k_{\text{el}}}$$

From a linear $\log_{10} C_P$ versus t plot we can obtain $T_{1/2}$ and therefore the elimination rate constant (k_{el}). k_{el} has the dimensions of h^{-1}, min^{-1}, or s^{-1} depending on whether $T_{1/2}$ is in hours, minutes or seconds respectively.

Clearance

Clearance concepts are considered to be more useful than $T_{1/2}$ for understanding drug elimination (reference 1). Thus, the emphasis in the remaining text will be on clearance rather than $T_{1/2}$.

Blood clearance (Cl_B) or plasma clearance (Cl_P) is the volume of blood or plasma cleared of drug in a unit time. It is obvious that clearance must be related in some way to the volume in which the drug is dissolved (volume of distribution, V_D) and the *rate* at which it goes out (i.e. related to $T_{1/2}$ or to the elimination constant k_{el}). In fact, clearance can be defined as the product of the volume of distribution and the elimination rate constant.

To illustrate the concept of clearance here are some simple examples:

Imagine a compartment of volume 100 ml in which there is initially 100 mg of drug. Suppose that elimination processes in the organs through which the biological fluid circulates completely remove the drug from 10 ml of this volume every minute. Figure 4 shows the minute-by-minute changes which occur.

In this example the clearance is constant ($10 \, \text{ml} \, \text{min}^{-1}$) whereas the amount of drug eliminated is reduced in each successive minute. If we plot the rate of drug eliminated

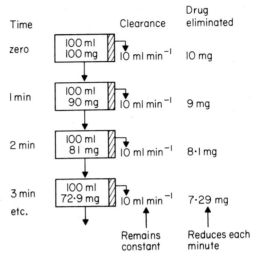

Figure 4

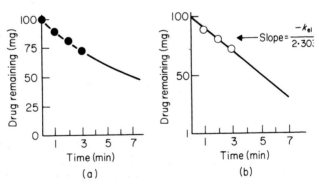

Figure 5

against time, or the drug remaining in the compartment against time we find an exponential (first-order) decline as shown in part (a) of Figure 5.

Plotted semi-logarithmically (part (b) of the figure) the data yield a straight line from which we obtain the elimination rate constant (k_{el}). (This works out at $0.1\,\text{min}^{-1}$.) We can show that the clearance ($10\,\text{ml min}^{-1}$) in this example is equal to the volume ($100\,\text{ml}$) multiplied by k_{el}. Clearance will be constant whilst k_{el} and volume remain unchanged. A change in clearance or volume will result in a change in k_{el}.

A number of factors can alter drug clearance such as renal or hepatic impairment and these will have a resultant effect on k_{el}. In reality the drug is not removed discretely from part of the volume *but the kinetics can be described as though it were.*

Let us now expand the example to the diagram below.

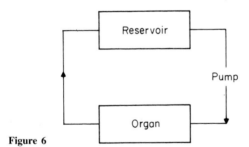

Figure 6

Let the total volume of the system be $100\,\text{ml}$. If the flow through the organ is $10\,\text{ml min}^{-1}$ and it removes (extracts) all of the drug, the same kinetic situation and values pertain as before. The diagram could be likened to the isolated perfused organ systems which are often used to study clearance.

Clearance

Plasma clearance is given by the relationship

$$Cl_P = V_D k_{el}$$

and the rate of elimination $= Cl_P \times C_P$.

If V_D is in ml and k_{el} in units of $\min^{-1}$, then Cl_P has the dimension $\text{ml}\,\text{min}^{-1}$.

Let us now assume that the organ does not remove all of the drug. For instance if only half of that which passes through is cleared there will be an organ flow of $10\,\text{ml}\,\text{min}^{-1}$ but a clearance of $5\,\text{ml}\,\text{min}^{-1}$. This partial clearance by the organ introduces the concept of extraction. If the volume remains constant it also follows that the elimination rate constant must halve.

Extraction

Unless the drug is administered locally, it has to be delivered to an organ by the blood. Therefore, the maximum rate of drug delivery to that organ is determined by the blood flow. If the organ takes up the drug from the blood to some extent, then *extraction* is said to occur.

By extraction we normally mean the irreversible removal of drug for example by excretion or metabolism. This results in a difference in drug-concentration between the blood flowing *into* and *out* of the organ. Thus, for example, we speak of *hepatic* or *renal extraction*.

The proportion of drug removed by a single transit of the

blood through the organ can be calculated from the ingoing and outgoing concentrations. This ratio is usually called the *extraction ratio* or *fraction* (E). Because the liver is often one of the major sites of drug elimination, the hepatic extraction ratios have been determined for many drugs of clinical importance. A good example of a high hepatic extraction drug is the β-blocker propranolol. Antipyrine is a low extraction drug.

The extraction by an organ can be calculated by the concentrations entering and leaving an organ.

$$E = \frac{C \text{ blood in} - C \text{ blood out}}{C \text{ blood in}}$$

Extraction is related to clearance by:

$$Cl = QE$$

where Q is the blood flow and E the extraction fraction or ratio (from 0 to 1)

The measurement of clearance

The simplified schemes shown so far would not apply for many drugs. Many are cleared by at least two routes, e.g. metabolism and renal excretion. However blood or plasma concentration data is all that is necessary to measure overall clearance. Because blood or plasma clearance is the product of the elimination rate constant and the volume of distribution, we would expect it to be closely related to the size or area of the concentration against time plot.

Clearance is the sum of individual clearance values. For example, plasma clearance (Cl_P) is the sum of metabolic clearance (Cl_M) and renal clearance (Cl_R) for a drug cleared by metabolism and renal excretion:

$$Cl_P = Cl_M + Cl_R.$$

A similar equation could be written for blood clearance. Or similarly, hepatic clearance could be the sum of clearance by metabolism and biliary clearance:

$$Cl_H = Cl_{BILE} + Cl_M$$

The hatched area (A) shown in the figure below is described as the area under the curve or AUC. Mathematically,

$$AUC_{0-\infty} = \int_0^{\infty} C_P \, dt.$$

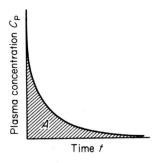

For intravenous bolus injection the clearance can be calculated from the relationship:

$$Cl_P = \frac{DOSE}{AUC}$$

Similarly blood clearance can be calculated from blood concentration data or from plasma data by knowing the partitioning of the drug between plasma and red cells over the range of concentrations measured from the relationship:

$$Cl_P = \frac{C_B (1 - \text{haematocrit})}{\text{Fraction of drug in plasma}}$$

or

$$Cl_P = Cl_B \left(\frac{C_P}{C_B} \right)$$

The relationship between clearance, DOSE and AUC is true whatever the route of drug administration. For routes other than intravascular, however, DOSE is equated with the fraction of the administered dose which is actually absorbed.

This relationship is particularly useful since clearance is independent of the type of pharmacokinetic model used. We will understand more of the pharmacokinetic model when we consider models with more than one compartment later.

Clearance, flow and extraction

We can modify the previous examples to the figure below.

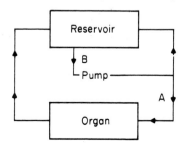

Figure 7

Let us suppose the organ receive 25% of the total pump output and removes all of the drug. The total volume (100 ml) is the same as before and the pump output is $40 \, \text{ml min}^{-1}$. Thus the organ receives $10 \, \text{ml min}^{-1}$ and since all of the drug is removed the clearance is also $10 \, \text{ml min}^{-1}$. The system can be likened to the human body with the pump the heart, the reservoir the various tissues and the organ the liver and kidneys. In each case the clearance by an organ is governed by extraction and flow. The flow to the organ is the fraction of the cardiac output that it receives. An extension of this system is found in Appendix 1 (physiological models).

Importance of site of administration

In the example above let us consider the site of administration of the drug. If we sample the perfusion fluid (blood) at site B and administer the drug at B we will see kinetics applicable to a model with a clearance of $10 \, \text{ml min}^{-1}$ and a volume of 100 ml. If we give the drug at site A however and sample at B we will see a major difference. Since the organ removes all of the drug, no drug will reach B. This example introduces the concept of the first-pass effect.

First-pass effects

Drugs which have high hepatic extraction ratios tend to exhibit marked *first-pass effects*. By this is meant that a large proportion of the drug being absorbed is removed before it can enter the general circulation. The blood flow from the gastrointestinal tract goes directly to the liver before returning to the heart and systemic circulation. Thus a substantial fraction of a drug being absorbed from the gastrointestinal tract may be metabolized by the liver or excreted into bile without ever reaching the rest of the body.

First-pass effects are important since they may explain why a drug can be potent when administered systematically and yet have no efficacy when given orally, despite having the characteristics necessary for absorption. When administered orally, the drug is removed in the first pass of the compound through the liver via the portal vein whereas, when administered systemically, only that fraction of the cardiac output directed through the liver can be cleared. First-pass effects need not be limited to the liver; the gastrointestinal tract itself, or the lung in the case of inhalation administration, could be sites of first-pass effects.

First pass

We can predict drugs which may undergo first-pass metabolism by the liver if we know the clearance of drug by this organ (Cl_H) and blood flow to the organ (Q_h). Knowing these values, we can calculate *extraction* from:

$$\text{Extraction } (E) = \frac{Cl_H}{Q_h}$$

The extraction ratio (E) or extraction is the fraction of drug removed from the blood during a single transit through the organ. The fraction of an oral drug (F_0) which reaches the systemic circulation is therefore given by:

$$F_0 = 1 - E$$

It is clear that drugs which have a high extraction will exhibit a marked *first-pass* effect.

Hepatic clearance (Cl_H) can be conveniently calculated from the blood (Cl_B) or plasma (Cl_P) clearance if we know the net contribution of Cl_H to the blood or plasma clearance or we know the sum of all other clearance processes (e.g. renal clearance, Cl_R). In the case of plasma clearance we also need to know the partitioning of the drug between red cells and plasma.

Thus, $$Cl_B = Cl_H + Cl_R + \ldots$$

If E is very high (i.e. approaches unity),

then $$Q_h \times E = Cl_H$$

becomes $$Q_h = Cl_H$$

and drug clearance by the liver depends on the hepatic blood flow (references 3 and 4).

The drugs which are subjected to first-pass effects by the liver are those of high extraction. Propranolol is a much researched example of such a drug. Variable kinetics are often found since small changes in the extraction may give rise to large changes in the fraction absorbed.

Intrinsic clearance (Cl_i) is the ability of an organ to clear a drug without flow limitation. The actual extraction of a drug can be calculated from:

$$E = \frac{Cl_i}{(Q + Cl_i)}$$

Thus clearance is given by:

$$Cl = \frac{QCl_i}{(Q + Cl_i)}$$

Where drugs have a high Cl_i in relation to Q the equation approximates to:

$$Cl = Q$$

as above where the specific example of the liver was chosen.

Where Cl_i is low relative to Q then the equation approximates to:

$$Cl = Cl_i$$

This concept is important since it relates blood flow and the metabolic capacity. Hepatic Cl_i can be calculated for drugs well absorbed from the gastro-intestinal tract by the equation:

$$Cl_i = \frac{DOSE}{AUC(oral)} = \frac{Cl}{F_0}$$

Area under the curve (AUC)

For a pharmacological response to occur in an organ or tissue different from the site of absorption, drug has to be carried there by the blood. It is therefore apparent that the intensity and duration of the tissue response is probably in most cases a function of the concentration and persistence of the drug in the blood or plasma.

Consider a typical plasma concentration versus time plot for a drug administered intravenously (see Figure 8).

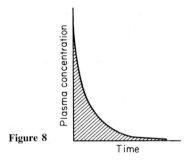

Figure 8

We would expect the size and duration of the biological response to be related in some way to the area under the curve (AUC), i.e. to the area of the hatched area shown in Figure 4 (above). Similarly, as outlined above, the AUC is also closely related to the clearance of the drug. A measure of this area can, therefore, be a useful index of the biological availability of the drug and a means of estimating its clearance.

It is important to understand that the area under the curve is not a direct *measure* of the dose, although it is obviously related. Consider the two areas shown in Figure 9.

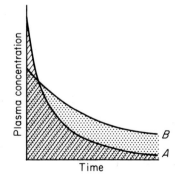

Figure 9

trations measured after an i.v. bolus dose. Note that a semi-logarithmic plot is shown. The experimental points lie on the solid line.

The plasma level decline can be divided into two phases, (1) and (2) in Figure 10.

The first phase (1) includes the distribution of drug from the central compartment, in this case the plasma and rapidly distributed tissues, into a second compartment. After a certain time period expressed here as X, equilibrium will be attained between the two compartments when they then behave essentially as one: the graph therefore moves into a log/linear phase (2) (line (b) in Figure 10). This log/linear phase represents elimination from the central compartment in equilibrium now, of course, with the second compartment. The slope of line (b) is used to determine a rate constant (β). This is calculated by a method analogous to the method for calculating k_{el} in the one-compartment model.

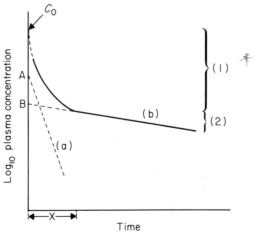

Figure 10

This rate constant β is usually referred to as a *hybrid rate constant* since it is a complex value related to several individual constants. It is the rate constant which governs the overall elimination rate of the drug in this case. The half-life which can be calculated from the rate constant β is often termed the *biological half-life*.

The zero-time intercept B (in Figure 10) represents the apparent concentration if the drug has been distributed instantaneously throughout both the central and second compartments. Thus, intercept B can be used to calculate an apparent volume of distribution (V_D). Other approaches are often used to calculate this value and other similar values. Line (a) in the figure results when C_P values which lie on line (b) are deducted from the real values of C_P. The slope of line (a) is used to determine another rate constant (α). The method of calculation is as before. This rate constant α is also a hybrid value and it is the constant which governs distribution of the drug into the second compartment.

Another zero-time intercept A (in Figure 10) can also be determined. If we add intercept A to intercept B we obtain C_0 which is the theoretical concentration of the drug in plasma at time zero. We can use this value to calculate the volume into which the drug is initially introduced (i.e. the volume of the central compartment V_C).

The hybrid rate constant, β, and the elimination rate constant, k_{el}, are closely related. In many cases elimination takes place only from the central compartment. Therefore, the rate of elimination at equilibrium is governed by the amount of drug in the central compartment rather than by the total amount of drug in the body (as is the case with the one-compartment model).

A frequent misconception is that the two phases always represent distribution (α) then elimination (β) as though the two occurred sequentially. Both processes occur at the same time and it is the relative rates of elimination and distribution that determine what the phases represent. For drugs of high clearance the initial α phase can represent a significant proportion of the drug elimination, with such drugs β can depend on rate of redistribution from peripheral compartments rather than elimination.

The concept of compartments

The diagram below illustrates one- and two-compartment models after an intravenous dose.

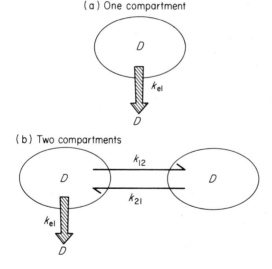

k_{12} and k_{21} are the rate constants which characterize the movement of drug from compartment 1 into compartment 2 and vice versa.

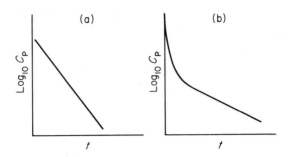

The two-compartment model is needed when there is a second more slowly equilibrating (deeper) compartment to be taken into account. Its presence is recognized by the shape of the $\log_{10} C_P$ vs time curve (part (b) above). Remember that a single-compartment model gives a linear semi-logarithmic plot (part (a) above).

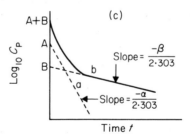

The figure (c) above shows the $\log_{10}$ plasma concentration versus time curve broken down to its contributing exponentials by the method of residuals (see Gibaldi & Perrier, 1975 or 1982, and example in Appendix 2).

Using the data we can calculate a number of useful parameters. By calculation of the slope of the linear terminal part of the curve (line b) we can determine the hybrid rate constant β. β is the rate constant from which the biological half-life of the drug can be calculated.

$$\text{Biological half-life} = \frac{0 \cdot 693}{\beta}$$

By extrapolation of line b to zero time we can calculate B, the intercept, and therefore an apparent volume of distribution V_D (sometimes referred to as V_B or $V_{D\beta}$) from

$$V_D = \frac{\text{DOSE}}{\text{B}}$$

or more usually by

$$V_D = \frac{Cl_P}{\beta}$$

By the process of residuals or exponential stripping (feathering) we can determine the hybrid rate constant α and the intercept value of this slope gives us A. With A and B known we can calculate a volume of the central compartment (V_C).

$$V_C = \frac{\text{DOSE}}{\text{A} + \text{B}}$$

Volume terms, however, are somewhat misleading with a two-compartment model since we do not usually wish to know the concentration present in the second compartment. We are normally more interested in the amount and this can be calculated without recourse to volume terms (see example in Appendix 2).

α and β are hybrid rate constants describing the curve and

$$C_P = Ae^{-\alpha'} + Be^{-\beta'}$$

Other relationships

$$\alpha + \beta = k_{12} + k_{21} + k_{el}$$

$$\alpha\beta = k_{21}k_{el}$$

We can, if we wish, calculate individual values for k_{el}, k_{21} and k_{12}:

$$k_{el} = \frac{\alpha\beta}{k_{21}} \quad \text{or} \quad \frac{A + B}{A/\alpha + B/\beta}$$

$$k_{21} = \frac{A\beta + B\alpha}{A + B}$$

$$k_{12} = \alpha + \beta - k_{21} - k_{el}$$

Plasma clearance is still obtained from the relationship

$$Cl_P = \frac{\text{DOSE}}{\text{AUC}_{0-\infty}}$$

We can conveniently obtain AUC for a drug given by intravenous bolus from the $\log_{10}$ plasma concentration versus time plot by the relationship:

$$\text{AUC} = \frac{A}{\alpha} + \frac{B}{\beta}$$

For a derivation of this and other relationships, see Gibaldi & Perrier 1975 or 1982.

The relative amounts that each phase contributes in terms of drug elimination can be estimated by comparing the relative areas:

$$\frac{A}{\alpha} \quad \text{and} \quad \frac{B}{\beta}$$

If $A/\alpha \ll B/\beta$ then the α phase is largely drug distribution. If $A/\alpha =$ or $> B/\beta$ a significant proportion of drug elimination takes place in this phase.

Other useful relationships include the following:

$$V_C = \frac{\text{DOSE}}{A + B}$$

$$V_{DSS} = V_C \left[(k_{21} + k_{12})/k_{21} \right]$$

where V_{DSS} is the predicted apparent volume of distribution at steady state. The apparent volume of the peripheral compartment V_P is given by:

$$V_P = \frac{V_C k_{12}}{k_{21}}$$

First-order and zero-order processes

Before we discuss intravenous infusions or oral dosing it is necessary to consider the difference between a *first-order* process and a *zero-order* one.

The exponential process described so far in which the amount of drug eliminated at any given time depends upon the *concentration* at that time is known as a *first-order* reaction. In mathematical terms, the exponent of the function is 1.

However, some processes are independent of the concentration of drug. The absorption of drug from a slow-release preparation, or a slow intravenous infusion of a drug are good examples. These are described as zero order. In some cases elimination may assume *zero-order* characteristics due to *saturation* of the elimination processes. The term *zero-order* is used because in mathematical terms the exponent of the function is zero; that is to say, the change in concentration

---

First-order and zero-order processes

The function:

$$D = D_0 \, e^{-k_{el}t}$$

is described as *first-order* since the exponent of the function is 1; that is to say, the change in concentration of D at a given time is dependent upon the concentration of D at that time.

Some processes, e.g. intravenous infusion, are said to be *zero-order* because the change in concentration is *independent* of the concentration, i.e.

$$\frac{-dD}{dt} = k_0$$

from which $D = k_0 t$, where k_0 is the zero-order rate constant. The graphs below compare zero- and first-order elimination.

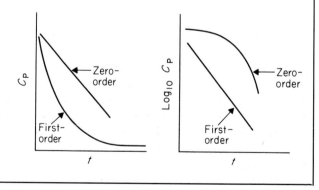

of the drug is independent of the concentration.

We will return to the significance of saturation and zero-order processes in elimination later in the text. For the present it is important to realize that first-order processes may become zero-order when high concentrations of drug are present.

Intravenous infusion

Consider a hypothetical situation where a drug is infused intravenously at a constant rate (i.e. a zero-order process), but *cannot be eliminated* either by metabolism or by excretion. It is reasonably obvious that the plasma concentration will rise steadily (e.g. linearly) until the infusion stops (Figure 11).

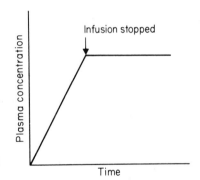

Figure 11

Let us now superimpose upon this the typical *concentration-dependent* (i.e. first-order) elimination which usually occurs. At first the elimination is very slow because the plasma concentration is low but it then increases until a maximum rate is reached which is equal to the infusion rate. We have now reached the steady-state level with a steady-state plasma concentration (C_{ss}).

At this point, as long as the same infusion rate is main-

tained, a constant plasma concentration will be maintained.
If the rate is increased then a new level will be set. As soon
as the infusion stops the plasma concentration begins to fall
in an exponential manner (See Figure 12).

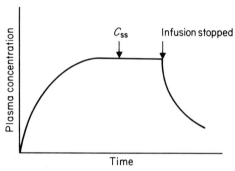

Figure 12

When we consider the process in this manner it is clear
that the shape of the rising part of the curve is governed by
the *elimination* process. It is possible to determine elimination
parameters (e.g. k_{el}) from the shape of this part of the
curve.

It is worth restating that the plasma concentration (and
the concentration of drug in other tissues in ready equilibrium
with plasma) will continue to rise until the *rate in* (rate of
drug infused) equals the *rate out* (rate of drug eliminated)
whereupon a constant concentration (steady state) is maintained. If either of the rates change a new steady-state level
will be achieved.

Since we can readily control the rate of infusion, pharmacokinetic analysis can allow us to set the appropriate rate to
achieve any desired steady-state plasma concentration.

The considerations which apply to an intravenous infusion
can also be applied successfully to a number of other important conditions in which drug is presented at a constant rate.
For example, this pharmacokinetic behaviour is exhibited

during inhalation of an anaesthetic gas, or during the appearance in blood of a drug from a slow release preparation (e.g. subcutaneous implant).

Intravenous infusion

Infusion is a zero-order process where k_0 is the rate constant for infusion, i.e. the rate at which the drug is infused. Thus, the amount of the drug infused at any time t is given by:

$$D = k_0 t$$

Given *first-order* elimination from plasma we have the situation shown in the following figure for a one-compartment model.

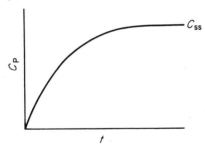

The rate of change of plasma concentration

$$\frac{dC_P}{dt}$$

gets less and less as the plateau value (C_{ss}) is approached. The shape of the curve is actually governed by the elimination characteristics of the compound.

The rate of elimination at any time t is given by:

$$C_P \text{ at time } t \times Cl_P$$

Since, at steady state, the rate of elimination (*rate out*) is equal to the rate of infusion (*rate in*) we have:

$$C_{ss} \times Cl_P = k_0$$

$$C_{ss} = \frac{k_0}{Cl_P}$$

If the clearance does not change, then the steady-state level is determined by the rate of drug infusion. For example, if we halve the rate of infusion, then C_{ss} will fall to half of its previous level.

The equation which describes the curve shown in the figure on page 37 involves k_0 and k_{el} and should show only one exponential function. Thus, the plasma concentration at any time t is given by

$$C_P = \frac{k_0}{V_D k_{el}} (1 - e^{-k_{el}t})$$

If the infusion is continued for long enough, the asymptotic plasma plateau concentration C_{ss} is obtained when

$$C_{ss} = \frac{k_0}{V_D k_{el}}$$

since $(1 - e^{-k_{el}t})$ approaches 1.

The amount of drug in the body at steady state is given by $C_{ss} \times V_D$. This is therefore equal to the ratio of the two rate constants.

Note that, since

$$C_{ss} = \frac{k_0}{V_D k_{el}} \quad \text{and} \quad Cl_P = V_D k_{el}$$

then, as shown above,

$$C_{ss} = \frac{k_0}{Cl_P}$$

The following useful relationships may be derived:

$$C_{ss}V_D = (1\cdot44)T_{1/2}k_0 \left(\text{since } T_{1/2} = \frac{0\cdot693}{k_{el}}\right)$$

and $t_x = -1\cdot44T_{1/2} \ln (1-x)$ where t_x is the time required to reach a designated fraction, x, of the plateau concentration or amount.

From this equation it follows that the fraction (x) of the plateau value which is attained after a given number of half-lives (N) is given by:

$$x = 1 - \text{antilog}_e \left(\frac{-N}{1\cdot44}\right)$$

e.g. after three half-lives ($N=3$) then $x = 0\cdot875$ (i.e. 87·5 per cent).

Partial infusion data

Sometimes the steady-state concentration C_{ss} is not even approached and only a partial infusion curve like the one in the figure below may be available for kinetic analysis.

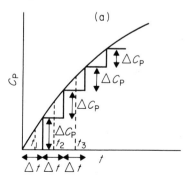

The slope of this partial curve is estimated at different time points (e.g. at t_1, t_2, t_3, etc. in the figure on page 39)

$$\frac{\Delta C_P}{\Delta t}$$

By plotting

$$\log_{10}\frac{\Delta C_P}{\Delta t}$$

against time we obtain a curve from which we may estimate kinetic parameters. The one- and two-compartment curves are shown in Figures (b) and (c) respectively (below).

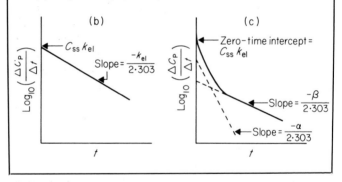

The single oral dose

When a single oral dose of a drug is given to someone there is usually a rise and then a fall in the plasma concentration as shown in Figure 13 on page 41.

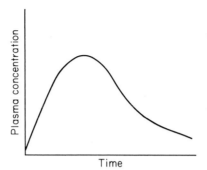

Figure 13

The rise in plasma concentration occurs during the *absorption* phase. The decline is sometimes said to be the elimination phase. However elimination starts immediately there is any drug in the plasma and absorption ends when no more drug reaches the circulation from the gastrointestinal tract. However, the time at which absorption ends is unlikely to coincide with the peak level since this only represents the time at which the <u>rate of drug absorbed equals the rate of drug eliminated</u>. <u>Thus during the rising part of the curve, the rate of absorption is greater than the rate of elimination. During the declining phase the rate of elimination is greater</u> than the rate of absorption.

We can represent the absorption phase in two ways: (i) as the disappearance of drug from the absorbing site (Figure 14(a) on page 42), or (ii) its corresponding curve, Figure 14(b) below, for the total of drug present in body at sites other than the absorption site or already eliminated.

We can see that curve B is an inverted reflection of curve A. It will be no surprise, therefore, that pharmacokineticists are able to calculate parameters for absorption as well as those for elimination from the total plasma concentration versus time curve.

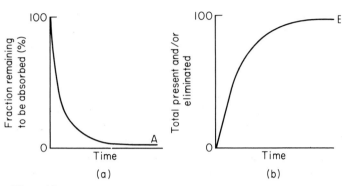

Figure 14

It is apparent that the absorption process of drugs may be complex. For example, due to saturation of absorptive capacity when the drug is highly concentrated in parts of the gastrointestinal tract, the process could have a *zero-order characteristic*. Another example is where the dissolution rate of the drug limits the rate of absorption. However, the zero-order characteristic may change to a *first-order* process while the concentration drops. What does this mean in practice if we measure plasma concentration at different times? Consider the two situations shown in Figure 15.

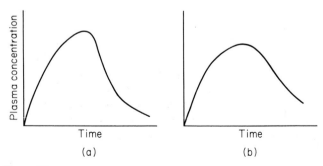

Figure 15

Part (a) of Figure 15 represents the case of *zero-order* absorption with *first-order* elimination for a single-compartment model, for example, as in an incomplete intravenous infusion. Part (b) of the figure represents the situation of *first-order* absorption with *first-order* elimination again for a single-compartment model. It is evident that there is not a great deal of difference between the two curves. A change from *zero-order* to *first-order* characteristics during the absorptive process would therefore result in a curve intermediate between the two. In practice, the course followed by most drugs fits *reasonably* well with *first-order* absorption, i.e. the decline in the amount of drug still to be absorbed follows the type of curve shown in Figure 14(a).

What information can be obtained from the measurement of plasma concentration at different times after a single oral dose? Other than the obvious advantage of being able to monitor the onset and duration of effective therapy and to predict potential toxic effects, we can obtain the following information from the observed pharmacokinetic behaviour.

1 Assuming *first-order* absorption and *first-order* elimination of the drug, we can calculate the absorption rate constant (k_{ab}) and the elimination rate constant (k_{el}). The mathematical solution to this problem must take into account whether the data fits better with a single-compartment or a two-compartment model. We also need to know whether $k_{ab} \gg k_{el}$ or vice versa.

2 The time at which the peak plasma concentration occurs is determined by the values of the two rate constants. The time to achieve this peak depends on this ratio.

3 The area under the plasma curve (AUC) is a useful measure of the amount of drug absorbed and eliminated. Therefore, the *biological availability* (*bioavailability*) of various formulations of the same drug may be compared.

Bioavailability and bioequivalence

Consider the three curves shown in Figure 16. Each of the three formulations A, B and C given at the same dose results in different peak plasma concentrations. However, the area under the curve for A and B is similar and therefore they are absorbed to a similar extent. Thus, they will be equally effective if the plasma concentration is not important for efficacy.

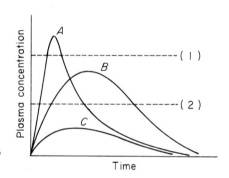

Figure 16

Consideration of the time at which the peak plasma concentration occurs shows that the rate constants of the two formulations are different. Since the elimination rate constant (k_{el}) is assumed to be the same in all cases (same drug), it is clear that the absorption rate constant (k_{ab}) is different, i.e. B is absorbed slower than A. Formulation C on the other hand gives a much lower area under the curve and therefore a lower proportion of the dose has been absorbed, resulting in lower availability and hence probably efficacy.

Other considerations could affect our choice of formulation. For example, the concentration indicated by (1) in Figure 16 could represent the plasma concentration at which an undesirable side effect occurs and the concentration indicated by (2) could represent the plasma concentration at which the drug is efficacious. Therefore, formulation *B* is superior to *A* on two factors even though the extent of absorption is comparable. Formulation *B* will have a longer duration of action than formulation *A* and will not exhibit the side effects seen with *A*. This simple example illustrates the importance of well-designed drug formulations in therapeutics.

The terms bioavailability and bioequivalence are not necessarily synonymous. We suggest that bioavailability has to do with the *amount* of drug present. *Bioequivalence* is also concerned with *efficacy*. Two formulations which have a similar bioavailability may yet differ significantly in efficacy. Equal bioavailability does not necessarily confer bioequivalence. Because of the ambiguity of meaning in published literature between the terms bioavailability, biological availability, and bioequivalence, it is always wise to define what is meant. Some authors prefer bioavailability to include a description of the *time course* as well as the total drug absorbed. In this case equal bioavailability does imply bioequivalence.

Other applications

The pharmacokinetic behaviour of a drug after a single oral dose applies equally well to the case of a single dose given by any means other than intravenously or intra-arterially. The mathematical considerations can be applied to the appearance of a metabolite of a drug in the plasma after an intravenous injection of the drug. Consider the plasma concentration−time curve in Figure 17.

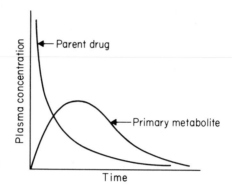

Figure 17

The parent drug can be likened to the drug present at the site of absorption in our previous examples. The primary metabolite concentrations follow a curve similar to that seen in plasma for the drug after oral absorption. Provided we have sufficient accurate data, we can build up a comprehensive knowledge of what is happening to all the parameters of drug absorption and metabolism.

Similar principles (but using more complex mathematics) may also be applied to consider the appearance of a metabolite after an oral dose of a drug or the appearance of a secondary metabolite produced from a primary metabolite after an intravenous dose of a drug.

A number of drugs require metabolic conversion to become active. To predict adequate dosage regimens for such drugs a knowledge of metabolite kinetics is required. It is outside the scope of this book to cover this in any depth and further reading on this topic is suggested (Gibaldi & Perrier, 1975 or 1982).

The single oral dose

First-order absorption with first-order elimination results in the typical plasma concentration versus time curve shown below.

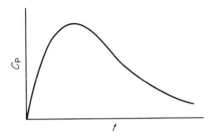

This curve is the result of two exponential processes, a fact reflected in the equation which describes the situation for the one-compartment model that we have already considered.

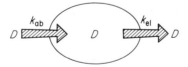

The equation involves both rate constants:

$$C_P = \frac{FD_0}{V_D} \frac{k_1}{k_1 - k_2} (e^{-k_2 t} - e^{-k_1 t})$$

F is the function of the dose D_0 which is absorbed. k_1 and k_2 are the two rate constants. However, from this data alone it is not possible to say whether $k_1 = k_{ab}$ or k_{el} and vice versa, since this equation has two solutions. For this reason (unless one goes by intuition, or V_D is known) it is necessary to determine k_{el} in a separate experiment using intravenous dosing.

In practice, many drugs are absorbed faster than they are eliminated and, in these cases, $k_1 = k_{ab}$, and $k_2 = k_{el}$.

Computer programs are available for curve fitting according to this model (and many other models). However, much information can also be obtained by graphical methods (see Appendix 2).

The general equation shown above has other applications. For example, in *metabolite production* we have:

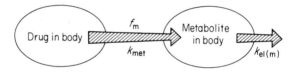

where f_m is the fraction of drug converted to metabolite, k_{met} is the rate constant for the production of the metabolite, and $k_{el(m)}$ is the rate constant for the elimination of the metabolite.

This is obviously similar to the processes we already know governing drug absorption and elimination (see figure below).

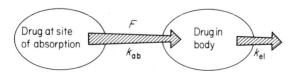

Thus, the equation given for absorption and elimination from a single compartment may also be used for metabolite production with appropriate substitutions of F by f_m and k_1 and k_2 by k_{met} and $k_{el(m)}$.

Equations describing first-order kinetics in various pharmacokinetic models

Exponential functions can be added together and therefore produce the general equations for the behaviour of drugs according to various pharmacokinetic models. For example, if we consider the equations which describe the time course of an i.v. bolus of a drug we find that for:

One-compartment: $C_P = C_0\, e^{-k_{el}t}$

Two compartment: $C_P = A\, e^{-\alpha t} + B\, e^{-\beta t}$

Three-compartment: $C_P = P\, e^{-\pi t} + A\, e^{-\alpha t} + B\, e^{-\beta t}$

where C_0, A, B, and P are constants. The experimental data are not usually sufficiently detailed or precise to allow separation of more than three compartments.

The same additive principle applies to absorption and elimination. Thus, for example, for a one-compartment model the equation:

$$C_P = \frac{FD_0}{V_D} \frac{k_{ab}}{(k_{ab} - k_{el})} \left(e^{-k_{el}t} - e^{-k_{ab}t}\right)$$

is seen to have the form:

$$C_P = Y\, e^{-k_{el}t} + Z\, e^{-k_{ab}t}$$

where the constant Y substitutes for

$$\left[\frac{FD_0 k_{ab}}{V_d(k_{ab} - k_{el})} \right]$$

and the constant $Z = -Y$.

Because elimination and absorption work in opposite directions an exponential absorption process will increase C_P whereas the elimination function decreases it.

As we might expect, the equation which describes first-order absorption and elimination from a two-compartment model has the form:

$$C_P = M\, e^{-\alpha t} + N\, e^{-\beta t} + R\, e^{-k_{ab}t}$$

where M, N and R are constants. Since $R\, e^{-k_{ab}t}$ is the function describing absorption, the constant R will have a negative value.

Repeated doses

Most drugs are administered more than once. Normally a patient will receive a course of treatment consisting of multiple applications of the drug. The frequency and size of each dose is described as a *dosage regimen*. We can alter significantly the efficacy of a drug by changing the dosage regimen.

Oral

Provided that oral doses are given sufficiently far apart in time they will behave independently, as in Figure 18, since each previous dose has been almost entirely eliminated.

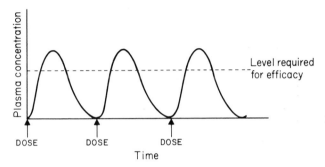

Figure 18

This is unsatisfactory if the level required for efficacy is as shown, and therefore the dosage regimen should be changed. The basic aim would be to give the drug several times a day with the deliberate intention of maintaining effective plasma concentrations. Thus, the second and subsequent doses would be given before the drug already present has had a chance to be cleared completely. What is the resulting shape of the plasma concentration versus time curve?

Consider the situation where the doses are *extremely small* but given at *very frequent* intervals. This is an approximation to the case of intravenous infusion (curve A in Figure 19). Thus, the plasma concentration would rise to a plateau, at which time the rate of elimination would equal the rate of absorption. In this extreme, hypothetical case the rate of accumulation is governed entirely by the size of these very small doses and their frequency. Absorption, then, has an

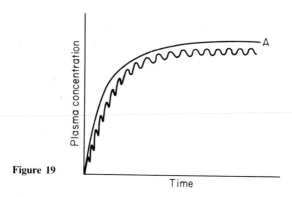

Figure 19

overall *zero-order* characteristic and the shape of the rising part of the curve reflects the elimination rate (as in the case of intravenous infusion).

In practice, discrete doses are given several times a day and result in a plasma concentration versus time curve having the general shape shown in Figure 20. The magnitude of the rises and falls which are superimposed upon the mean overall increase depends upon the size and frequency of doses and upon the elimination rate.

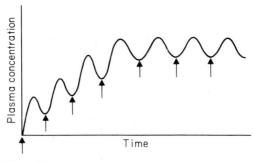

Figure 20

Nevertheless, after repeated dosing, a plateau concentration (steady-state level) will be achieved. The plateau will have maximum and minimum values in keeping with the frequency of dosing. The overall average concentration will be determined by the rate of drug administration (i.e. size of individual doses multiplied by the frequency) and the rate of elimination. The average plateau concentration will be achieved when the *rate of drug intake equals the rate of elimination*.

As in the case of an intravenous infusion, if we change the rate of drug administration, then a new average plateau concentration will be achieved. For example, if we double the size of each dose, or we increase the frequency at which individual doses are administered twofold, then we would see a twofold increase in average steady-state level.

Intravenous

Repeated intravenous dosing is somewhat similar to repeated oral dosing but less complex since the absorption phase is removed. Thus, given sufficiently far apart, doses behave independently (Figure 21); given sufficiently close together

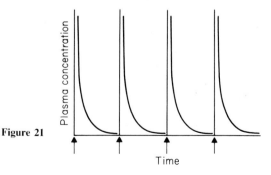

Figure 21

we reach the infusion situation which, in practice, gives the situation shown in Figure 22. Once again, a plateau is reached when the rate of drug entry equals its rate of elimination.

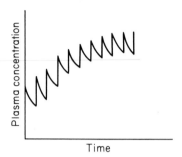

Figure 22

These examples of repeated dose kinetics emphasize the importance of explaining to a patient why he or she must follow the recommended dosage regimen. Many medicines are rendered ineffective or toxic because of failure to do this. This also indicates why dosage regimens should be altered when there is a lower plasma clearance giving rise to elevated steady state concentrations (e.g. in elderly or renally compromised patients).

General considerations

These apply to both repeated oral and repeated intravenous doses. With certain assumptions (e.g. whether it is a one- or a two-compartment model), it is possible to calculate the plateau maximum, minimum and average values for any given dose size and frequency if the elimination rate constant (k_{el}) is known or can be measured. This information is valuable for adjusting dosage for individual patients and for predicting effective dosage regimens in general. The equations needed are given by Gibaldi & Perrier (1975 or 1982).

Repeated doses

A useful relationship for predicting the average steady-state plasma concentration ($\bar{C}_{ss}$) which could be reached after repeated doses is:

$$\bar{C}_{ss} = \frac{F(\text{DOSE})}{Cl_P T}$$

where DOSE is the individual dose, and T is the time interval between doses. F is the fraction of each dose which is available. This relationship is model independent. Notice the similarity between this and the equation governing intravenous infusion (page 38).

'Loading' doses

Since a single dose of a drug may be insufficient to achieve efficacious plasma concentrations, we may have to wait until after the administration of three or four doses before the patient begins to respond to treatment. In a case of serious illness this wait may be undesirable.

To achieve an effective plasma concentration as rapidly as possible, a particularly large initial dose may be given. This is called a 'loading' dose, and the following simplified example shows how it works.

Consider an antibiotic drug which is given in doses of 400 mg *intravenously* at four-hourly intervals. Assume that the plasma half-time $T_{1/2}$ is four hours. Table 1 shows the progress up to a steady-state situation when the amount eliminated in four hours is 400 mg which equals the amount injected.

Table 1

Time (h)	Dose given (mg)	'Dose' still left in body (mg)	Total drug present (mg)
0	400	0	400
4	400	200*	600
8	400	300	700
12	400	350	750
16	400	375	775
20	400	388	788
Plateau i.e. steady state reached	400	400	800

* Since $T_{1/2} = 4$ hours.

Now consider what happens when an initial 'loading' dose of 800 mg is given and followed up with four-hourly doses of 400 mg (Table 2; $T_{1/2} = 4$ hours).

Table 2

Time (h)	Dose given (mg)	'Dose' still left in body (mg)	Total drug present (mg)
0	800	0	800
4	400	400	800
8	400	400	800

Thus, the 'plateau' or steady-state situation in this case is achieved immediately instead of taking more than 20 hours as it does when regular equal-sized doses are given. This may be of considerable advantage in a life-theatening situation.

Excretion of drugs in urine

The collection of plasma samples may cause distress to a patient or be impossible for other reasons. However, it is frequently possible to collect serial urine samples after drug administration. The measurement of the drug or metabolites which appear and the rate at which they appear can also be used to obtain pharmacokinetic information. In some cases, both urine and plasma samples may be collected to give additional information.

Consider the case of a drug given intravenously which is eliminated unchanged from plasma only by urinary excretion (assuming a one-compartment model). The appearance of the drug in the urine will be a reflection of the disappearance from the plasma or from the body (Figure 23).

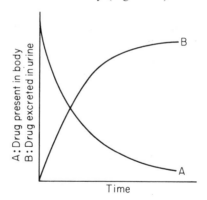

Figure 23

If the logarithm of the amount of drug either remaining or excreted is plotted against time, we get the lines shown in Figure 24. The resulting plot of the amount of drug still present in the body (A) is linear and, from this, the half-life ($T_{1/2}$) of the drug and the elimination rate constant (k_{el}) may be calculated. Plot B is less convenient for calculating a rate constant as it follows a curve.

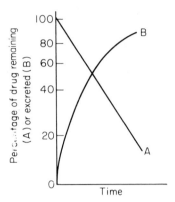

Figure 24

It is actually more convenient to plot the logarithm of the amount of drug *remaining to be excreted*. In this previous example we have assumed that *all* of the drug is excreted in the urine and, therefore, the graph of the amount remaining to be excreted in the urine against time is identical to the graph of the amount of drug present in the body against time. Both can be used to determine the elimination rate constant (k_{el}). It can also be shown that a plot of the logarithm of the amount of drug remaining to be excreted against time is governed by k_{el} irrespective of the fraction of the drug which is excreted in urine. The example at the end of the book (Appendix 2, Exercise 9) will illustrate the concept more clearly.

Excretion of drugs in urine after an intravenous dose

For a one-compartment model the amount of drug found in urine (after an i.v. dose D_0) is given by the following relationship:

$$D_{\mathrm{u}} = \frac{k_{\mathrm{u}}D_0}{k_{\mathrm{el}}}\,(1 - e^{-k_{\mathrm{el}}t})$$

where D_{u} is the *cumulative* amount of unchanged drug excreted to time t, k_{u} is the rate constant for the first-order excretion process and D_0 and k_{el} are the dose and elimination rate constants respectively.

The amount ultimately excreted (D_{u}^{∞}) is therefore:

$$D_{\mathrm{u}}^{\infty} = \frac{k_{\mathrm{u}}D_0}{k_{\mathrm{el}}}$$

since $(1 - e^{-k_{\mathrm{el}}t})$ approaches 1. Thus,

$$D_{\mathrm{u}} = D_{\mathrm{u}}^{\infty}(1 - e^{-k_{\mathrm{el}}t}).$$

Therefore, the elimination rate constant may be determined from the urinary excretion data. For convenience, we plot the amount *remaining to be excreted* rather than the amount excreted. The amount remaining to be excreted is defined as:

$$(D_{\mathrm{u}}^{\infty} - D_{\mathrm{u}}) = D_{\mathrm{u}}^{\infty} - D_{\mathrm{u}}^{\infty}(1 - e^{-k_{\mathrm{el}}t})$$
$$= D_{\mathrm{u}}^{\infty}\,e^{-k_{\mathrm{el}}t}$$

Therefore, if we plot $\log_{10}(D_{\mathrm{u}}^{\infty} - D_{\mathrm{u}})$ versus time we find:

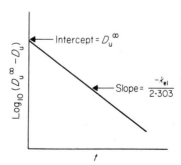

The elimination rate constant is obtained from the slope of the line.

k_u can be obtained from:

$$D_u^\infty = \frac{k_u D_0}{k_{el}}$$

The method is sometimes called the sigma minus ($\Sigma-$) method. In practice, it requires collection of urine samples until no further drug is excreted.

The method can be used irrespective of the number of compartments. It is found that the urinary excretion reflects the plasma data and can be used to determine α and β, for example, in a two-compartment model.

Incomplete urinary excretion data

Sometimes incomplete urinary excretion data is available which makes the former method impossible. In this case an estimate of D_u^∞ and k_{el} can be obtained by plotting

$$\log_{10} \frac{\Delta D_u}{\Delta t}$$

against t (Figure (b)). Where $\dfrac{\Delta D_u}{\Delta t}$ values are the slopes of the D_u versus t plot (Figure (a)).

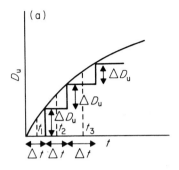

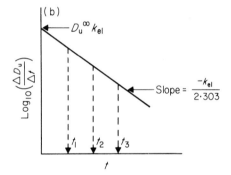

The semi-log plot will reflect the plasma elimination. The slope of the straight line (in the case of a one-compartment model) is

$$\frac{-k_{el}}{2 \cdot 303}$$

and the zero-time intercept is $D_u^\infty k_{el}$. Thus, an estimate of kinetic parameters can be made.

Capacity-limited processes

The clinical significance of capacity-saturated elimination

Zero-order processes in the elimination of drugs are often of importance. *Zero-order* elimination occurs because the processes of elimination other than glomerular filtration have a limited capacity. The drug concentration cannot be raised indefinitely to cause a corresponding rise in the rate of elimination. Sooner or later the elimination is saturated. The level at which this occurs largely determines the dose of drug which can be tolerated without accumulation occurring. If, however, the elimination capacity has been saturated but therapy with the drug is still continued, then accumulation, and therefore probably toxicity, rapidly ensues.

Instead of an exponential decline in the plasma concentration, zero-order elimination is characterized by a straight line in a linear plot (Figure 25a) which, in the semi-logarithmic form, gives a convex curve (Figure 25b). We can contrast these zero-order plots with the first-order plots described earlier and illustrated in parts (c) and (d) of Figure 25.

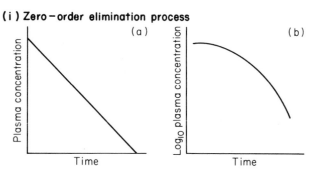

(i) Zero – order elimination process

Figure 25 a and b

(ii) First-order elimination process

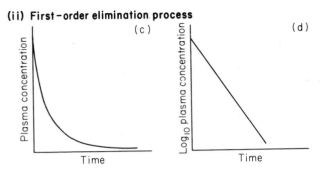

Figure 25 c and d

Consider two intravenous doses of a drug: a low dose which is eliminated by a first-order process, and a high dose which, because the elimination routes are saturated, will exhibit *zero-order* characteristics until the level falls sufficiently. The $\log_{10}$ plasma concentration versus time plots are shown in Figure 26. Once the concentrations of drug have fallen sufficiently, the elimination processes will no longer be saturated and elimination will return to first-order following the high dose.

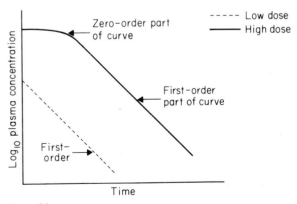

Figure 26

If we measure the decline in plasma concentration with time for a series of intravenous doses of a drug which exhibits capacity-saturated elimination we can determine the threshold dose at which this occurs. For the example shown in Figure 27, zero-order characteristics are first seen between the 20- and 30-mg doses. The threshold dose therefore lies somewhere between these two doses. A knowledge of this threshold value is clinically important if the therapeutic dose is of a similar order.

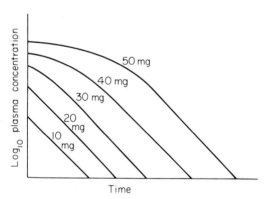

Figure 27

A knowledge of capacity limited processes is important for understanding toxicity and drug accumulation. Alcohol exhibits zero-order elimination even at quite low doses and therefore accumulation and resulting inebriation can occur rapidly if its consumption is continued.

Saturation with any drug may occur in metabolism, biliary excretion or active renal excretion. One or more of these processes may be involved.

Other capacity-limited processes

We have already considered briefly how absorption may change from *zero-order* to *first-order*. We mentioned that the initial zero-order process could be due to saturation of the absorptive process.

Drugs with a marked first-pass effect often exhibit a greatly increased bioavailability at high doses. This is because the hepatic extraction (often metabolism) of the compound has a limited capacity (see reference 5). This is clinically important because the dose−response or dose−toxicity relationship will not be linear. A modest increase in an oral dose could result in a disproportionate increase in efficacy or unfortunately in some cases, toxicity.

In the case of a drug exhibiting non-linear kinetics, intravenous infusion will eventually produce steady state blood or plasma concentrations provided that the infusion rate is less than the maximal rate of elimination (V_{max}). The nearer the rate of input approaches V_{max} then the more dramatic will be the effect upon the steady state level. This is illustrated in Figure 28 (page 68). In Figure 28 the curve is normalized. The steady state level is expressed as a multiple of K_m (defined as the blood or plasma concentration at half maximal rate of elimination) and the infusion rate is expressed as a fraction of V_{max}. Another consequence of nonlinear kinetics is that (unlike the linear case) the time needed to reach steady state increases dramatically as the infusion rate approaches V_{max}.

The same principles apply to repeated i.v. bolus, or oral doses in a manner analogous to the linear case.

The model independent parameter of clearance and AUC are useful for dealing with non-linear kinetics. Thus clearance is still equal to DOSE/AUC. However, in this case clearance is not a constant and AUC is not proportional to dose. The concept of compartments still applies in non-linear cases although the mathematics are complex. Estimates of V_{max} and K_m can sometimes be obtained graphically (a simple example is included in exercise 10) but more usually by computer methods.

Capacity-limited elimination

At high concentrations of drug in the plasma the elimination process (i.e. metabolism, excretion) may become saturated resulting in zero-order elimination. In some cases zero-order elimination is important even at therapeutic drug levels. We can understand what is happening in mathematical terms by reference to the Michaelis–Menten expression for enzyme kinetics (reference 6) because elimination processes conform closely to this expression.

$$v = \frac{V_{max}\,(S)}{K_m + (S)}$$

V_{max} and K_m are enzyme constants (kinetic parameters) governing the maximum velocity (V_{max}) and the 'affinity' of the substrate S for the enzyme (K_m). If we consider the substrate concentration (S) to be proportional to the plasma concentration, and v to be the rate of drug elimination, then rate of drug elimination is proportional to

$$\frac{V_{max}\,C_P}{K_m + C_P}.$$

At low plasma concentration $C_P \ll K_m$

$\therefore$ $C_P + K_m$ is approximately equal to K_m

∴ rate of drug elimination is proportional to

$$\frac{V_{max} \, C_P}{K_m}$$

Since V_{max} and K_m are constants, the rate of drug elimination is proportional to the plasma concentration at *low* plasma concentrations.

On the other hand, at very high plasma concentration $C_P \gg K_m$

∴ $$C_P + K_m \approx C_P$$

and rate of drug elimination is proportional to

$$\frac{V_{max} \, C_P}{C_P} \text{ (i.e. } \propto V_{max})$$

∴ *rate of drug elimination is a constant.*

For i.v. infusion when Michaelis–Menten kinetics apply steady state is reached when the rate of input (K_0) equals the rate of elimination v. Thus:

$$K_0 = v = \frac{V_{max} \, C_{ss}}{(K_m + C_{ss})}$$

Expressing K_0 as a fraction (x) of V_{max} we have:

$$\frac{K_0}{V_{max}} = x = \frac{C_{ss}}{(K_m + C_{ss})}$$

From which:

$$C_{ss} = \frac{K_m x}{(1 - x)}$$

(i.v. infusion concepts can also be readily applied to steady state oral kinetics)

Since K_m is defined as the blood or plasma concentration at half maximal rate of elimination we can express C_{ss} in terms of K_m. A graph of x against C_{ss}/K_m (C_{ss} as a multiple of K_m) is shown in Figure 28.

The increasing deviation from linearity as K_0 approaches V_{max} is illustrated.

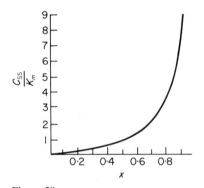

Figure 28

Another useful relationship is the following:

$$\text{AUC} = C_0[(C_0/2) + K_m/V_{max}]$$

where C_0 is the plasma concentration at time 0.

Protein binding

Clearance, volume of distribution and half life may all depend on protein binding. By protein binding we normally mean a reversible association of the drug to the proteins of the blood or tissues. With blood binding the single most important protein is albumin although other proteins such as α-1 acid glycoprotein assume importance with certain classes of compounds. Binding is normally due to ionic and hydrophobic forces between drug and protein. Such reversible binding must not be confused with irreversible binding which is a drug clearance process. Reversibly bound drug will be in equilibrium with the free drug, the amount bound depending on the affinity of the drug for a particular protein. The blood or tissues will therefore contain both free and bound drug. It is a widely accepted view that only free drug is available for clearance, distribution or to exert pharmacological and toxic effects. Most analytical methods do not discriminate between bound and free drug, measuring only the total. This is not of importance in many cases where the degree of binding by blood and tissues remains constant over the concentration range encountered after drug administration. The pharmacokinetics are adequately determined by measurement of total drug. Protein binding is of importance where the degree of binding is variable over the range of concentrations encountered after administration. With these drugs the degree of binding decreases with concentration, i.e. a disproportionate amount of free drug is available for distribution, clearance, pharmacological or toxic effects. In such cases the pharmacokinetics of the free drug can be usefully investigated. This requires separation of free from bound drug either during the assay procedure or by extrapolation from the results of other experiments (e.g. *in vitro* equilibrium dialysis).

Protein binding

The diagrams illustrated on page 29 can be extended to include bound and free drug:

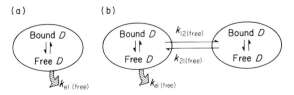

Note that only free drug is available for clearance, elimination and distribution. We can rewrite conventional equations for free drug rather than total thus:

$$Cl_p(\text{free}) = \frac{\text{DOSE}}{\text{AUC } 0-\infty(\text{free})} \text{ (cf. page 18)}$$

or at steady state:

$$C_{ss}(\text{free}) = \frac{K_0}{Cl_p(\text{free})} \text{ (cf. page 38)}$$

and using the ratio of free to total drug f:

$$f \times C_{ss}(\text{Total}) = \frac{K_0}{Cl_P(\text{free})}$$

where f represents the free fraction in plasma.

The last two equations show that during intravenous infusion if drug binding decreases with increasing concentration (f increases) then $C_{ss}(\text{total})$ will no longer increase proportionally with K_0. $C_{ss}(\text{free})$ will however still increase in proportion.

Conclusion

What is the relevance of pharmacokinetics? As we have seen, the discipline is an attempt to quantify what happens to drugs in the body and therefore has very important applications, in therapeutics, toxicology, pharmaceutics and pharmacology. We hope that some of these applications will have become clear to you during your reading of this text. We also hope that you have become sufficiently interested in the subject to want to read further. A short bibliography is given to assist you.

Although not covered in this text, there are a number of aspects of drug disposition (i.e. what happens to a drug in the body) in which pharmacokinetic considerations are important. These include, for example, the factors affecting absorption, pathways of metabolism, tissue binding and the mechanisms of biliary and renal excretion of drugs. Variations in these and other parameters can result in marked differences in the pharmacokinetic behaviour of drugs between species and even between individuals. Since drugs are normally administered to patients rather than to healthy people it is worth noting that the disease itself can create significant variations in the pharmacokinetics of a drug (references 7 and 8). Similarly, as mentioned the age of the patient may be of importance (references 9 and 10).

Finally, pharmacokinetic analysis of drug behaviour is most useful when it is based on good data. The importance of obtaining sufficient data points of appropriate accuracy cannot be over-stressed (see Appendix 3). The value of pharmacokinetic parameters which are estimated are only as good as the data on which they are based. Pharmacokinetic analysis, like statistical analysis, can, however, be abused or can lead the unwary investigator into error (reference 11). The best guide, as always, is common sense.

Appendices

1: Physiological models

In conventional compartmental pharmacokinetic analysis 'compartments' are mathematical concepts which fit the data closest. They may or may not relate to real compartments or volumes. Physiological modelling attempts to include real tissues and volumes. A simple example is shown in Figure 29.

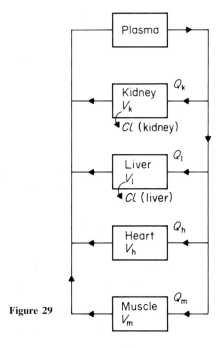

Figure 29

(V_k, V_l, V_h etc. are the volumes of the various tissues and Q_k, Q_l, Q_h etc. their blood flows. Cl(kidney) and Cl(liver) are the clearances by clearing organs.)

Other compartments (fat etc.) may be added as required. The rate of change of the plasma concentration at any time depends upon the rate of removal and the rate of return from the tissues. The rate of change of tissue concentration at any time depends upon the rate of delivery and the rate of removal either by return to the plasma or by elimination from the particular tissue.

Differential equations are written to describe these changes and solved by the use of computers. The mathematics involved are beyond the scope of this text. Potentially the method yields more detailed information than the usual compartmental model in which the parameters may not be directly related to the physiology of the animal. From this type of model it is easy to see how disease states (e.g. decreased renal function; Q_k or Cl(kidney) impaired) alter the overall kinetics. (See reference 12.)

2: Pharmacodynamics

It is important to stress that pharmacokinetics is but one link in the relationship between administered dose and biological effect. A simple scheme illustrates this:

Administered dose $\rightarrow$ Pharmacokinetic effect $\rightarrow$
Pharmacodynamic phase $\rightarrow$ Drug effect

The pharmacokinetic phase has been covered within the contents of the book. This phase encompasses the processes that affect the concentration of drug circulating in the plasma (or blood). The pharmacodynamic phase describes those processes that link the concentration of drug in the circulation with the biological effect. This phase can be conceptually viewed by the following relationship, assuming the drug acts reversibly at a receptor or similar drug target:

$$C_P \rightleftarrows C_r \rightleftarrows \text{drug}-\text{receptor complex} \rightarrow \text{drug effect}$$

where C_r is the local drug concentration at the receptor.

When examining the relationship between administered dose and drug effect, a plot of drug effect versus logarithm of the administered dose will frequently yield a sigmoidal curve. At very low doses no effect is discernible, at high doses the effect reaches a maximum. The intermediate region of this plot, covering approximately 20–80% of the maximum drug effect, is linear. This relationship can be improved by substituting the log of the plasma concentration for the administered dose, thereby removing variations due to the pharmacokinetic phase. Such variations may reflect differences in bioavailability or clearance between individuals. This simple substitution is particularly appropriate in cases where C_P, C_r and the drug–receptor complex are in rapid reversible equilibrium.

Many drug targets are present in sites distinct from the circulation and the drug may take time to diffuse or distribute to its site of action. In other cases the kinetics of the drug's disassociation with the receptor may be slower than the drug's elimination from the circulation. These effects, where C_P, C_r and the drug–receptor complex slowly or do not apparently equilibrate, can all be modelled using compartmental principles similar to those described for the pharmacokinetic phase. This modelling process is termed concentration-effect analysis or pharmacodynamic modelling and extensive reviews are available (see reference 13). Whilst this book has concentrated on the pharmacokinetic phase, the pharmacodynamic phase is equally important. Unless the plasma (or blood) concentration-effect relationship, and the factors affecting it, is known (pharmacodynamic phase), then pharmacokinetics is powerless to predict drug effect.

3: Exercises

The exercises are designed to illustrate the concepts discussed in the text. We have used simulated data for clarity and convenience although an attempt has been made to provide a background to each example to illustrate the value of pharmacokinetic analysis. Expert mathematical knowledge is not required to answer the questions set, only semi-logarithmic paper, and a calculator, log tables or a slide rule. The answers can be found after Appendix 2 on pages 98 to 100.

Graphical methods

The subject of pharmacokinetics is becoming an increasingly complex one. To keep pace with these complexities, more sophisticated methods of handling data have been developed using both digital and analogue computers. Graphical methods, however, still offer a rapid method of processing data and can be adapted to yield various types of information. The plotting of data is, in itself, a method of analysis and much is gained by graphical portrayal of data with careful thought given to the time- and concentration-scales that are used. In these exercises examples of some of these techniques are explained. Some simple semi-logarithmic paper is appended to this book. This will enable you to obtain approximate answers to the exercises. More accurate results will be obtained however, with commercially available paper.

Graphical methods can be used for *resolving* or for *predicting*. Graphical methods are most useful when applied to first-order kinetic processes when they are generally based upon two main concepts: (1) that a semi-logarithmic plot of an exponential function (of form $A\ e^{-\alpha t}$) is linear, and (2) exponentials are additive (the principle of superposition). Thus, the method of 'residuals' described in several of these exercises consists of resolving a semi-logarithmic curve into a series of straight lines (i.e. the opposite of 'superposition'). The reader is encouraged to develop such methods for himself. Further examples where graphical methods can be applied include the following:

1 The prediction of plasma concentrations resulting from any number of doses by the principle of superposition.

2 The determination of the amount of drug in the peripheral compartment of a two-compartment model.

3 To plot the amount of metabolite in plasma with time if k_m and $k_{el(met)}$ are known and one-compartment kinetics are followed.

4 Evaluation of urinary data for a drug obeying two or more compartment kinetics.

5 For recognizing zero-order processes by studying the shape of the plot. For example, plot semi-logarithmically plasma concentration data for a drug undergoing zero-order absorption into a one-compartment system. Now apply the method of 'residuals'. In this case it is found that the 'absorption' residual line is convex on the semi-log plot but *linear if replotted on ordinary graph paper*. This indicates that the absorption process is zero order. The shape of plots for drugs undergoing zero-order elimination can be found in the text on pages 62 and 64.

Most of the equations required can be found in Gibaldi & Perrier (1975 or 1982).

Exercise 1: Intravenous bolus — one-compartment model

Phenytoin sodium (300 mg) was administered intravenously to a patient with epilepsy. The plasma concentration of phenytoin was then monitored to determine the pharmaco-kinetic behaviour of the drug and to help in establishing an optimum oral dosage regimen for this patient. The results obtained were as follows:

Time (h)	Plasma concentration C_P (μg ml^{-1})
5	4·70
10	3·65
15	3·05
20	2·40
30	1·45
40	0·93
50	0·61

1 Plot $\log_{10} C_P$ against time and C_P against time. For convenience, use semi-log paper for the $\log_{10}$ plot (e.g. Chartwell, log 3 cycles × mm, reference 5531 or graph paper at the back of the book).

2 From the slope of the $\log_{10}$ plot calculate the half-life of phenytoin, and from the half-life calculate the elimination rate constant (k_{el}) using the relationship:

$$k_{el} = \frac{0·693}{T_{1/2}}$$

The units of k_{el} will be in hours^{-1}.

3 Extrapolate the straight line in the $\log_{10}$ plot back to zero time and determine C_0. Using this value calculate the volume of distribution from the relationship; DOSE $= C_0 \times V_D$. The volume of distribution will be in ml; however, it is more convenient to quote this as litres. Remember to convert the dose to μg.

---

78 *Exercises*

4 Calculate the plasma clearance of phenytoin from the relationship:

$$Cl_P = V_D \times k_{el}$$

The units will be litres hour^{-1} since V_D is in litres and k_{el} in hours^{-1}.

Exercise 2: Further analysis using the data given in Exercise 1

Calculate the area under the plasma curve by using each of the following methods:

1
$$AUC_{0-\infty} = \frac{C_0}{k_{el}}$$

2
$$AUC_{0-\infty} = \frac{DOSE}{Cl_P}$$

3 the trapezoid method (Gibaldi & Perrier 1975 or 1982).

This third method simply divides the curve of the C_P against time plot into a series of small straight lines. The average concentration of each of these straight lines is then calculated and multiplied by the time between the two points to give the area under the curve; i.e. in the figure below, AUC_{A-B} = average value of $C_P \times$ time.

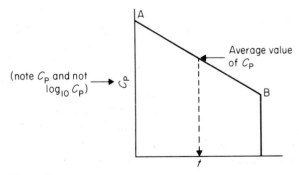

(note C_P and not $\log_{10} C_P$)

Figure 30

If this process is repeated for the whole curve, the total area under the curve can be calculated. In the example given in Figure 31 this is:

$$AUC_{A \to D} = (A' \times a) + (B' \times b) + (C' \times c).$$

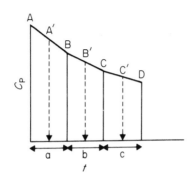

Figure 31

The simplest method is to use the experimentally determined time points in the table given in Exercise 1. In this example, however, two further values are required for the complete AUC (i.e. $AUC_{0-\infty}$). These are a value of C_P for zero time (i.e. C_0 from the $\log_{10} C_P$ vs time plot) and a practical value for $t = \infty$. This value, again taken from the $\log_{10} C_P$ vs time plot for example, could be when 99 per cent of the drug has been eliminated (i.e. after about 100 hours). Commonly, however, the AUC is extrapolated to infinity by the relationship (C_{P_t}/k) where C_{P_t} is the concentration at the last time point ($0 \cdot 61 \, \mu g \, ml^{-1}$ in this example) and k is the rate constant represented by the slope at this instant in time (equal to k_{el} in this example).

Notice that the first two methods give identical results and that the result of method 3 is very similar. Methods 1 and 2 are much more rapid. The trapezoidal method is important, however, when it is not possible to use simple linear relationships as will be seen in later exercises.

Exercise 3: Oral dose — one-compartment model (1)

Phenytoin (300 mg) was subsequently given orally to the same patient and the following plasma concentrations recorded.

Time (h)	Plasma concentration C_P (μg ml^{-1})
1	0·65
2	2·00
5	3·55
10	4·05
15	3·60
20	3·20
30	2·00
40	1·20
50	0·75

1 Plot $\log_{10} C_P$ against time and C_P against time. For convenience use semi-log paper for the $\log_{10}$ plot.

2 Notice the rise and then subsequent fall of the plasma concentration with time. Also observe that the terminal slope of the curve is log-linear. From this portion of the curve calculate $T_{1/2}$ and k_{el} as described previously. Are these values the same as those calculated in Exercise 1?

3 Calculate the absorption rate constant (k_{ab}) by the method of residuals.

Extend the log-linear line to zero time (intercept Z). For a one-compartment model with first-order absorption the zero time intercept is

$$Z = \frac{F \times \text{DOSE} \times k_{ab}}{V_D(k_{ab} - k_{el})}$$

where F is the fraction of the oral dose which is absorbed.

Having extended the log-linear line to time zero, read off and list the values on this line at each of the time points from zero time until the attainment of the log-linear phase.

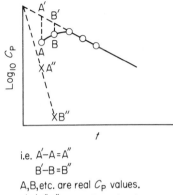

i.e. A′–A = A″
   B′–B = B″
A,B,etc. are real C_P values.

Figure 32   A′,B′,A″,B″ are projected values.

Subtract the real measured plasma concentrations from these projected values. You will now have a third series of apparent C_P values. Plot these on the same $\log_{10}$ plot and draw a straight line through the points.

The zero time intercept of this second straight line will also be Z. From the slope of this second straight line calculate a half-life ($T_{1/2}$ for absorption) and k_{ab} from

$$\frac{0 \cdot 693}{T_{(1/2)ab}}$$

4 Calculate the $AUC_{0-\infty}$ described by the plasma concentration after the oral administration of the drug by two methods:

i the trapezoid method as before,
ii using the relationship:

$$AUC_{0-\infty} = \frac{Z}{k_{el}} - \frac{Z}{k_{ab}}$$

5 Compare the above AUC value with that obtained after an i.v. dose (Exercise 2). What is the value of F from the relationship:

$$F = \frac{AUC_{oral}}{AUC_{i.v.}}$$

6 Having determined F, calculate the plasma clearance of phenytoin after an oral dose using the relationship:

$$Cl_P = \frac{F \times DOSE}{AUC_{oral}}$$

Is the value the same as that after the intravenous dose?

7 Using your values of Z, k_{ab}, k_{el} and F, calculate V_D from the relationship:

$$V_D = \frac{F \times DOSE \times k_{ab}}{Z(k_{ab} - k_{el})}$$

Also calculate V_D from the relationship:

$$V_D = \frac{Cl_P}{k_{el}}$$

Are the two values the same and the same as the volume of distribution after the i.v. dose?

Exercise 4: Oral dose — one-compartment model (2)

The patient was subsequently treated with oral phenytoin at 100 mg three times a day. After a certain period of treatment during which the epilepsy was moderately controlled, an attempt was made to improve therapy. The patient was therefore given another brand of tablet with a different formulation. Instead of improving, the patient's epilepsy became worse. Further plasma estimations were therefore obtained after a single test dose of 300 mg of the new tablets. Ideally,

Time (h)	Measured plasma concentration C_P ($\mu g\,ml^{-1}$)	Projected concentration due to 'residual' drug ($\mu g\,ml^{-1}$)	Projected concentration due to test dose ($\mu g\,ml^{-1}$)
-2	2·20		
0 (test dose)	2·00	2·00	0
1	2·20	1·90	0·30
2	2·53	1·83	0·70
5	2·60	1·60	1·00
10	2·70	1·25	1·45
15	2·55	1·00	1·55
20	2·23	0·80	1·43
30	1·63	0·50	1·13
40	1·20	0·32	0·88
50	0·85	0·20	0·65
60	0·55	0·13	0·42
80	0·23	0·05	0·18

there should be a 'wash out' period during which treatment is stopped before the test dose but this is not always practicable or advisable. In this case notice that the patient had a plasma concentration of $2 \cdot 2\,\mu g\,ml^{-1}$ 2 hours before the test dose was given. This was due to continuous prior therapy with phenytoin.

1 Plot $\log_{10} C_P$ against time.

2 It is first necessary to distinguish between the change in concentration due to the residual phenytoin and that due to the test dose.

Notice that the plasma concentration was $2 \cdot 2\,\mu g\,ml^{-1}$ 2 hours before the test dose and that this declined to $2 \cdot 0\,\mu g\,ml^{-1}$ by zero time. This appears to be falling with a half-life of about 15 hours if we assume a log-linear relationship. This half-life is the same as that found previously for this patient. Therefore, draw a straight line which has a slope equivalent to $T_{1/2} = 15$ hours, intercepting at $2.0\,\mu g\,ml^{-1}$ (zero time). The values which lie on this line represent the amount of phenytoin present from previous doses. Deduct the values at each time point from the actual values. The differences represent the phenytoin from the test dose.

N.B. In case you find this step somewhat complicated we have done this for you in the table on page 83. Check that you get similar values.

3 Having generated a list of C_P values which reflect phenytoin resulting from the test dose (i.e. a list similar to the last column in the table), calculate the elimination and absorption rate constants for this brand of tablet as in Exercise 3. Note that it can be done on the same semi-log plot as before.

4 Compare the values of k_{ab} and k_{el} with those obtained in Exercise 3.

5 Calculate the $AUC_{0-\infty}$ as in Exercise 3.

6 Calculate F as before.

7 Calculate the plasma clearance.

8 What is the cause of the lack of therapeutic control?

9 Predict the average steady-state plasma concentration $(\bar{C}_{ss})$ which would be achieved in this patient taking 100 mg three times daily. Use the relationship:

$$\bar{C}_{ss} = \frac{F \cdot (DOSE)}{Cl_P \times T}$$

where T is the time between doses (i.e. assume 8 hours) and Cl_P is the value you have already determined. Does the value you have calculated agree with the residual plasma concentrations shown in the table?

10 Finally, calculate the $\bar{C}_{ss}$ which would be predicted if the patient were put back on the original tablets.

Note: Phenytoin is a very important drug in clinical medicine. Its pharmacokinetic behaviour has been studied extensively and is more complex than has been depicted in these examples. It is a drug which exhibits characteristic Michaelis—Menten kinetics (see Exercise 10).

Exercise 5: Continuous intravenous infusion (1)

A patient who had undergone major surgery required a slow intravenous infusion of aminocaproic acid to control haemorrhage. The infusion was given for 24 hours at a rate of $1\,g\,h^{-1}$. Plasma concentrations of aminocaproic acid were monitored and yielded the results given in the table below.

Time (h)	Plasma concentration C_P ($\mu g\,ml^{-1}$)
2	37
4	65
6	83
8	97
12	113
16	122
20	128
24	130

1 Plot the data on to ordinary graph paper and semi-logarithmic paper. Notice the steady-state concentration (C_{ss}) and when this is achieved.

2 Calculate k_{el} by the method of residuals. To do this, calculate $C_{ss} - C_P$ (for time points from the start of infusion to attainment of steady state).

Plot $\log_{10}(C_{ss} - C_P)$ against time. From the straight line calculate k_{el} using the relationship:

$$k_{el} = \frac{0 \cdot 693}{T_{1/2}}$$

3 Determine the plasma clearance of the drug and its volume of distribution from the steady-state concentration and the rate of infusion using the relationships:

$$C_{ss} = \frac{\text{rate of infusion}}{Cl_P} \text{ and } Cl_P = k_{el} \times V_D$$

Exercise 6: Continuous intravenous infusion (2)

There may be occasions when it is not possible nor desirable to continue an intravenous infusion to steady state, and yet an estimate of the pharmacokinetic behaviour of the drug is required. This could apply, for example, during emergency infusions with potentially dangerous drugs such as procainamide or propanolol. An estimate of kinetic parameters may be obtained in such cases by the following graphical method. As an example we have used only the first four values given in Exercise 5.

Time (h)	C_P (μg ml^{-1})	ΔC_P	Δt(h)	$\frac{\Delta C_P}{\Delta t}$	Average time points
0	0				
		37	2	18·5	1
2	37				
		28	2	14·0	3
4	65				
		18	2	9·0	5
6	83				
		14	2	7·0	7
8	97				

1 Now plot

$$\log_{10} \left(\frac{\Delta C_P}{\Delta t} \right)$$

against time (using the 'average' time points between the two points). Use semi-logarithmic paper for convenience.

2 A log-linear plot results. The slope of this line is

$$\left(\frac{-k_{el}}{2 \cdot 303} \right).$$

Thus, $T_{1/2}$ and therefore k_{el} may be determined.

3 The zero time intercept is equal to $C_{ss} \times k_{el}$. C_{ss} may therefore be predicted even though the steady state has not yet been reached. Compare your values of C_{ss} and k_{el} with those found in Exercise 5.

Exercise 7: Continuous intravenous infusion (3)

It is necessary to give a continuous infusion of benzylpenicillin to a patient with meningitis. Benzylpenicillin pharmacokinetic behaviour corresponds to a one-compartment model. The plasma half-life of this antibiotic is 30 minutes and the volume of distribution corresponds to the volume of the extracellular fluid.

1 Calculate the rate of infusion which is required to maintain the plasma concentration at $20 \, \mu g \, ml^{-1}$. The steady-state plasma concentration is given by the relationship:

$$C_{ss} = \frac{k_0}{Cl_P}$$

where Cl_P equals $V_D \times k_{el}$ for a one-compartment model. Assume that $V_D = 15$ litres (extracellular fluid).

Calculate k_{el} from

$$T_{1/2} = \frac{0.693}{k_{el}}$$

and obtain k_0 in mg min^{-1}.

2 How long will it take to reach 90 per cent of the steady-state level with this rate of infusion?

Using semi-logarithmic graph paper draw a straight line with a slope corresponding to a half-life of 30 minutes. Make the zero time intercept equal to $20\,\mu$g ml^{-1}. 90 per cent of the steady-state plasma concentration will be $18\,\mu$g ml^{-1}.

Since the vertical axis on the graph is equal to $(C_{ss} - C_P)$ you just need to read off the time when your line reaches $2\,\mu$g ml^{-1} (i.e. $20 - 18$).

3 Calculate a suitable initial (loading) dose to allow an almost immediate plasma concentration of $20\,\mu$g ml^{-1}.

There are several ways of looking at this problem. One way would be to calculate the amount in the body which is represented by a plasma concentration of $20\,\mu$g ml^{-1}. The drug required is given by the relationship:

$$D = C_P \times V_D$$

This amount of drug would need to be injected as a rapid intravenous bolus followed immediately by the rate of infusion you have already calculated. Such a measure could be vital to this patient's treatment.

4 Calculate the plasma concentration at 30 and at 60 minutes assuming that this loading dose is given and followed immediately by the infusion. Remember that exponentials can be added together. Thus, to calculate the actual plasma concentration 30 minutes after an initial dose followed immediately by the infusion, you have to add two values. One value is the plasma concentration at $t = 30$ resulting from the initial dose (remember the half-life is 30 minutes).

The second value is for the plasma concentration at time $t = 30$ resulting from the infusion. This can easily be obtained from the semi-log graph you have already drawn. Do the same calculation for $t = 60$ minutes.

Exercise 8: Intravenous bolus dose — two compartment model

A patient was given an intravenous injection of 50 mg of pethidine for post-operative pain. The kinetics of this drug are obviously of importance since pain relief is closely related to plasma concentration. The following data were obtained:

Time (h)	Plasma concentration C_P (μg ml^{-1})
0·5	0·42
1·0	0·29
1·5	0·22
2·0	0·18
2·5	0·15
3·0	0·125
4·0	0·096
6·0	0·060
8·0	0·038
10·0	0·024

1 Plot C_P against time using semi-logarithmic paper for convenience. Notice that the resulting plot is not linear over its whole length.

2 Notice, however, that the terminal part of the plot is log-linear. Extrapolate this line back to zero time to give B. From the slope of the line obtain β from the relationship

$$T_{1/2\beta} = \frac{0\cdot693}{\beta}$$

List a series of values lying on this line at early time points (e.g. at 0·5, 1·0, 1·5, 2·0, 2·5, 3·0 hours). Deduct each of these extrapolated values from the actual C_P value. Now plot the resulting differences (or residuals) semi-logarithmically. This procedure yields a second straight line from which A and α may be calculated in a manner analogous to B and β. You should now have values for A, α, B, β.

3 The results indicate that pethidine obeys two-compartment kinetics.

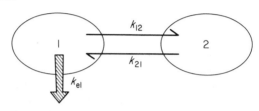

Figure 33

You may now solve the model for pethidine completely using the following relationships:

(a)
$$\text{Biological half-life} = \frac{0\cdot693}{\beta}$$

(b)
$$k_{21} = \frac{A\beta + B\alpha}{A + B}$$

(c)
$$k_{el} = \frac{\alpha\beta}{k_{21}} \quad \text{or} \quad \frac{A + B}{(A/\alpha) + (B/\beta)}$$

(d)
$$k_{12} = \alpha + \beta - k_{21} - k_{el}$$

(e)
$$Cl_P = \frac{\text{DOSE}}{\text{AUC}}, \quad \text{where} \quad \text{AUC} = \frac{A}{\alpha} + \frac{B}{\beta}$$

By applying the method of residuals we have resolved a biexponential decline into two separate exponential processes. Each of these (corresponding to α and β lines) is represented by a log-linear plot. In Exercise 1 we showed that the AUC of a log-linear plot was equal to

$$\frac{\text{intercept}}{k_{\text{el}}}.$$

Thus, the AUC of each residual is given by

$$\frac{A}{\alpha} \quad \text{or} \quad \frac{B}{\beta}$$

respectively and the

$$\text{total AUC}_{0-\infty} = \frac{A}{\alpha} + \frac{B}{\beta}$$

4 Prepare a plot using the available data which describes the amount of drug in the central and second compartments. The data are at present in terms of plasma concentration. This can be converted to total drug in the central compartment by multiplying by the volume of the central compartment which is given by

$$\frac{\text{DOSE}}{A + B}.$$

The data have been calculated below; check that your values are in agreement.

Time (h)	Plasma concentration ($\mu g\,ml^{-1}$)	Drug in central compartment (mg)
0·5	0·42	32·8
1·0	0·29	22·6
1·5	0·22	17·2
2·0	0·18	14·0
2·5	0·15	11·7
3·0	0·125	9·8
4·0	0·096	7·5
6·0	0·060	4·7
8·0	0·038	3·0
10·0	0·024	1·9

If we plot these new data using semi-logarithmic paper, we will obtain a graph which can be broken down into A, B, α and β as before (see Figure 34(i)). Notice that (A + B) is a new value and it is equal to the DOSE; α and β are the same values as before. The curve for the total drug in the central compartment (X_C) is described by $X_C = A\ e^{-\alpha t} + B\ e^{-\beta t}$. The equation governing the drug in the second compartment (X_P) is:

$$X_P = \frac{k_{12} \times \text{DOSE}}{\alpha - \beta}\ (e^{-\beta t} - e^{-\alpha t})$$

It should be apparent that

$$\left(\frac{k_{12} \times \text{DOSE}}{\alpha - \beta}\right)$$

is an intercept value and can be calculated from the values already determined. If we calculate this value and mark the point as a zero time intercept on our graph of drug in the central compartment (Figure 34(ii)), we can draw lines from this point parallel to the α and β slopes we already have (Figure 34(iii)). Now it is possible to calculate by the method of residuals the difference between our newly drawn lines and plot the resultant curve (Figure 34(iv)). The new curve will describe the amount of drug present in the second compartment with time. Note the example illustrated is a general one, and not the specific example detailed in the question.

Exercise 9: Urinary excretion — one-compartment model

Kanamycin is an antibiotic which is excreted unchanged mainly in urine. A patient was therefore treated with this antibiotic for a urinary tract infection. It is obviously of importance to understand the kinetics of the drug, particularly

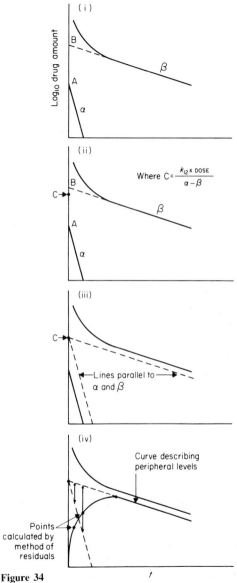

Figure 34

with respect to its urinary concentration. The following results were obtained after an intramuscular dose of 500 mg.

Time of urine sample collection (h)	Amount of drug (mg) in each sample	Cumulative amount (D_u)
0–0·5	73	72
0·5–1·0	63	135
1–2	90	225
2–4	113	338
4–8	84	422
8–24	28	450

1 Calculate $(D_u^\infty - D_u)$ which represents drug remaining to be excreted, and plot $\log_{10}(D_u^\infty - D_u)$ against t. Notice that the value of t for each value of D_u will be the time at which the urine collection was stopped since our values of $(D_u^\infty - D_u)$ (drug remaining in body) apply to this time. Since the rate of excretion has declined to a very low value by 24 hours, D_u^∞ can be assumed to be approximately equal to 450 mg (i.e. 90 per cent of the dose administered).

2 From the log-linear plot calculate k_{el} using the relationship:

$$T_{1/2} = \frac{0.693}{k_{el}}$$

Notice that the zero time intercept is 450 mg (i.e. D_u^∞). Calculate the urinary excretion rate constant (k_u) from the relationship

$$k_u = \frac{D_u^\infty}{\text{DOSE}} \times k_{el}$$

Exercise 10: Michaelis−Menten kinetics

As indicated in the note at the end of exercise 4, phenytoin is generally found to exhibit Michaelis−Menten kinetics. This exercise demonstrates one simple method for estimating the parameters V_{max} and K_m from plasma concentration data. The following results were obtained after a single oral dose of phenytoin (500 mg).

Time (h)	Plasma concentration C_P (mg litre^{-1})
10	10·4
20	8·2
30	6·5
40	4·8
60	2·4
80	1·0
100	0·42

1 Plot $\log_{10} C_P$ against time.

2 Extrapolate the terminal linear part of the curve back to zero time and estimate the intercept C'.

3 Estimate the zero time intercept of the actual data (C_0) from this determine V_d by:

$$\frac{\text{DOSE}}{C_0}.$$

4 K_m is estimated from the relationship:

$$K_m = \frac{C_0}{\ln{(C'/C_0)}}$$

5 Determine the half-life of the straight line you have drawn. From this calculate

$$K' = \frac{0·693}{T_{1/2}}$$

6 Estimate V_{max} from:

$$V_{max} = K'K_m$$

7 V_{max} is in units of concentration so multiply by V_d to give units of drug. Units are h^{-1} so multiply by 24 to give maximum daily amount that can be eliminated.

Exercise 11: Intrinsic clearance and blood flow

1 A development compound was administered at a dose level of $10\,mg\,kg^{-1}$ to a dog by intravenous administration. The area under the blood curve (AUC) was calculated to be $650\,min\,.\,\mu g\,ml^{-1}$. Calculate the systemic blood clearance (Cl_b) using the equation:

$$Cl_b = \frac{\text{DOSE}}{\text{AUC}}$$

Note: express your answer normalized to body weight (kg^{-1}).

2 The compound is cleared solely by metabolism in the liver (hepatic clearance). The liver blood flow is assumed to be $40\,ml\,min^{-1}\,kg^{-1}$. Calculate the hepatic extraction (E) using the equation:

$$Cl_b = QE$$

3 What fraction of dose would reach the systemic circulation if the drug was administered orally and it were completely absorbed from the gastrointestinal tract? ($F = 1 - E$).

4 Calculate the intrinsic clearance of the compound (Cl_i) using the equation:

$$Cl_i = \frac{QE}{(1 - E)}$$

Note: This equation reduces to $Cl_i = Cl_b/F$ from 2 and 3 above.

5 When administered chronically the compound induces its own metabolism. Over a 10 day dosing period the AUC value for the first dose of $20\,\text{mg}\,\text{kg}^{-1}$ given orally was $800\,\text{min}\,.\,\mu\text{g}\,\text{ml}^{-1}$. By the tenth dose the AUC for the dose declined to $460\,\text{min}\,.\,\mu\text{g}\,\text{ml}^{-1}$. Calculate the intrinsic clearance for the beginning and end of the study. Since:

$$Cl_i = \frac{Cl_b}{F} \quad \text{and} \quad Cl_b = \frac{F\,\text{DOSE}}{\text{AUC(oral)}}$$

after oral administration therefore:

$$Cl_i = \frac{\text{DOSE}}{\text{AUC(oral)}}$$

Is the value at the beginning of the study in agreement with that calculated previously?

6 Using the value for intrinsic blood clearance at the end of the study calculate the expected systemic clearance of the compound from the equation:

$$Cl_b = Q\left[\frac{Cl_i}{(Q + Cl_i)}\right]$$

7 At a single oral dose of $40\,\text{mg}\,\text{kg}^{-1}$ the compound increased cardiac output. The liver blood flow was increased to $50\,\text{ml}\,\text{min}^{-1}\,\text{kg}^{-1}$. There was no change in the intrinsic clearance value which remains at that previously calculated after intravenous administration. What effect, using the equations above, will this have on the fraction of drug reaching the circulation and on the systemic blood clearance? Will the AUC of the compound be greater or smaller if no blood flow change occurred? (see 5 above).

Answers—

Note: Answers obtained by graphical methods are approximations and you may see small differences between your answers and these.

Exercise 1

2 $T_{1/2} = 15\,\text{h}$
  $k_{el} = 0.046\,\text{h}^{-1}$
3 $V_D = 50$ litres
4 $Cl_P = 2.3$ litres h^{-1}

Exercise 2

1 and 2 $130\,\mu\text{g ml}^{-1} \times$ hours
3 $130\,\mu\text{g ml}^{-1} \times$ hours, using $0.61/0.046$ for the last time-point and $C_0 = 6\,\mu\text{g ml}^{-1}$

Exercise 3

2 $T_{1/2} = 15\,\text{h}$
  $k_{el} = 0.046\,\text{h}^{-1}$
3 $T_{(1/2)ab} = 3.5\,\text{h}$
  $k_{ab} = 0.2\,\text{h}^{-1}$
  $Z = 7.8\,\mu\text{g ml}^{-1}$
4 AUC = 130, 133 (by trapezoid method)
5 $F = 1.0$
6 $Cl_P = 2.31$ litres h^{-1}

Exercise 4

3 Absorption $T_{1/2} = 6.9\,\text{h}$
  $k_{ab} = 0.1\,\text{h}^{-1}$
  $k_{el} = 0.046\,\text{h}^{-1}$
5 AUC = $65.2\,\mu\text{g ml}^{-1} \times$ hours
6 $F = 0.5$
7 $Cl_P = 2.3$ litres h^{-1}
8 Only half of the phenytoin is available and the rate of absorption is also much reduced. Ineffective plasma concentrations are reached.

9 $C_{ss} = 2 \cdot 7\,\mu\text{g ml}^{-1}$ when $F = 0 \cdot 5$
   $C_{ss} = 5 \cdot 4\,\mu\text{g ml}^{-1}$ when $F = 1 \cdot 0$

Exercise 5
2 $T_{1/2} = 4\,\text{h}$
   $k_{el} = 0 \cdot 17\,\text{h}^{-1}$
3 $Cl_P = 7 \cdot 7\,\text{litres h}^{-1}$
   $V_D = 45\,\text{litres}$

Exercise 6
2 $T_{1/2} = 4\,\text{h}$
   $k_{el} = 0 \cdot 17\,\text{h}^{-1}$
3 $C_{ss} = 127\,\mu\text{g ml}^{-1}$

Exercise 7
1 $k_0 = 6 \cdot 93\,\text{mg min}^{-1}$
2 $100\,\text{min}$
3 $300\,\text{mg}$
4 $20\,\mu\text{g ml}^{-1}$
   $20\,\mu\text{g ml}^{-1}$

Exercise 8
2 $\text{DOSE} = 50\,\text{mg}$
   $A = 0 \cdot 4\,\mu\text{g ml}^{-1}$
   $B = 0 \cdot 24\,\mu\text{g ml}^{-1}$
   $\alpha = 1 \cdot 39\,\text{h}^{-1}$
   $\beta = 0 \cdot 23\,\text{h}^{-1}$

3 (a) Biological half-life $= 3\,\text{h}$
   (b) $k_{21} = 0 \cdot 66\,\text{h}^{-1}$
   (c) $k_{el} = 0 \cdot 48\,\text{h}^{-1}$
   (d) $k_{12} = 0 \cdot 47\,\text{h}^{-1}$
        $\text{AUC}_{0-\infty} = 1 \cdot 33\,\mu\text{g ml}^{-1} \times \text{hours}$
   (e) $Cl_P = 37 \cdot 6\,\text{litres h}^{-1}$

Exercise 9
2 $k_{el} = 0 \cdot 347 \, h^{-1}$
   $k_u = 0 \cdot 312 \, h^{-1}$

Exercise 10
3 $V_d = 42$ litres
4 $K_m = 12 \, mg \, litre^{-1}$
5 $K' = 0 \cdot 044 \, h^{-1}$
6 $V_{max} = 0 \cdot 53 \, mg \, litre^{-1} h^{-1}$
7 Maximum daily dose $= 530 \, mg$

Exercise 11
1 $Cl_b = 15 \cdot 4 \, ml \, min^{-1} kg^{-1}$
2 $E = 0 \cdot 385$
3 $F = 0 \cdot 615$ (61·5%)
4 $Cl_i = 25 \, ml \, min^{-1} kg^{-1}$
5 Beginning 25, end $43 \cdot 5 \, ml \, min^{-1} kg^{-1}$
6 $Cl_b = 20 \cdot 8 \, ml \, min^{-1} kg^{-1}$
7 $F = 0 \cdot 667$ (66·7%), $Cl_b = 16 \cdot 7 \, ml \, min^{-1} kg^{-1}$, AUC would remain unchanged as F increased but Cl_b also increased with increasing blood flow.

4: The importance of collecting adequate data

Pharmacokinetic modelling is based upon the data generated. For example, the figure below illustrates two sets of plasma concentration data obtained in the same patient on different occasions. The patient was given the same dose of drug intravenously on each occasion. The data are plotted semi-logarithmically.

Note that:
1 On the first occasion the drug kinetics appear to fit a one-compartment model because early samples were not collected.

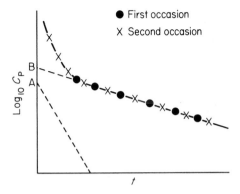

Figure 35

2 The clearance on the first occasion would be estimated from DOSE/AUC where AUC = B/k_{el}, and on the second occasion from DOSE/AUC where AUC = $A/\alpha + B/\beta$, since β for the two-compartment model and k_{el} have the same numerical value (because the slope is the same) the plasma clearance of the drug will be overestimated on the first occasion due to not collecting samples early enough.

Exercise 1 described one-compartment pharmacokinetic behaviour for i.v. phenytoin. However, if we had measured the plasma concentrations over the first few hours we would have discovered that the drug appears to obey two-compartment kinetics.

Bibliography

General reading

Pharmacokinetics

1 Gibaldi M. & Perrier D. (1975, 1982) *Pharmacokinetics: Drugs and the Pharmaceutical Sciences, Vol. 1*. (1st and 2nd editions — both are useful) Marcel Dekker, New York.
2 Bowman W.C. & Rand M.J. (1980) *Textbook of Pharmacology*, 2nd ed. Blackwell Scientific Publications, Oxford. Chapter 40 is particularly pertinent and is an excellent follow-up to this book.
3 Rowland M. & Tozer T.N. (1980) *Clinical Pharmacokinetics, Concepts and Applications*. Lea & Febiger, Philadelphia.

General principles of drug disposition

1 Goldstein A., Aronow L. & Kalman S.M. (1974) *Principles of Drug Action. The Basis of Pharmacology*, 2nd ed. John Wiley, New York.
2 Smith S.E. & Rawlins M.D. (1976) *Variability in Human Drug Response*, 2nd ed. Butterworth, London.
3 Curry S.H. (1980) *Drug Disposition and Pharmacokinetics — with a consideration of pharmacological and clinical relationships*, 3rd ed. Blackwell Scientific Publications, Oxford.
4 Routledge P.A. & Shand D.G. (1979) Presystemic drug elimination. *Ann. Rev. Pharmacol. Toxicol.* **19**, 447−68.
5 Wilkinson G.R. (1987) Clearance approaches in pharmacology. *Pharmacol. Rev.* **39**, 1−47.

References

1 Perrier D. & Gibaldi M. (1974) Clearance and biologic half-life as indices of intrinsic hepatic metabolism. *J. Pharmacol. Exp. Therap.* **191**, 17.
2 Wilkinson G.R. & Shand D.G. (1975) A physiological approach to hepatic drug clearance. *Clin. Pharm. & Therap.* **18**, 377.
3 Shand D.G., Kornhauser D.M. & Wilkinson G.R. (1975) Effects of route of administration and blood flow on hepatic drug elimination. *J. Pharmacol. Exp. Therap.* **195**, 424.

4 Benet L.Z. (1978) Effect of route of administration and distribution on drug action. *J. Pharmacokinet. Biopharm.* **6**, 559.

5 Raafaub J. & Dubach U.C. (1975) On pharmacokinetics of phenacetin in man. *Europ. J. Clin. Pharmacol.* **8**, 261.

6 Metzler D.E. (1977) *Biochemistry, the Chemical Reactions of Living Cells*, pp. 305−6. Academic Press, London.

7 Levy G. (1977) Pharmacokinetics in renal disease. *Am. J. Med.* **62**, 461.

8 Klotz U. (1976) Pathophysiological and disease-induced changes in drug distribution volume: pharmacokinetic implications. *Clin. Pharmacokinet.* **1**, 204.

9 Crooks J., O'Malley K. & Stevenson I.H. (1976) Pharmacokinetics in the elderly. *Clin. Pharmacokinet.* **1**, 280.

10 Rane A. (1976) Clinical pharmacokinetics in infants and children. *Clin. Pharmacokinet.* **1**, 2.

11 Fell P.J. & Stevens M.T. (1975) Pharmacokinetics — uses and abuses. *Europe. J. Clin. Pharmacol.* **8**, 241.

12 Rowland M. (1984) Physiologic pharmacokinetic models: relevance, experience, and future trends. *Drug met. Rev.* **15**, 55.

13 Holford H.N.G. & Sheiner L.B. (1981) Understanding the dose effect relationship: clinical application of pharmacokinetic-pharmacodynamic models. *Clin. Pharmacokinet.* **6**, 249.

Semi-logarithmic graph paper

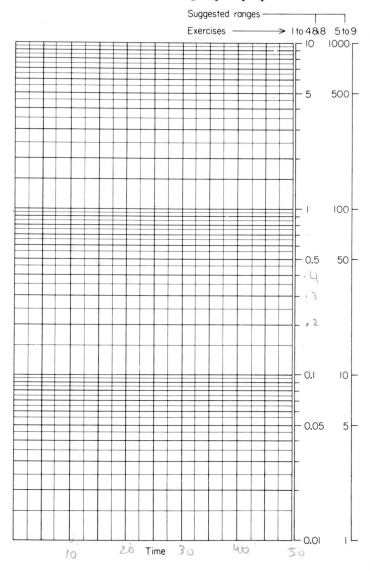

Suggested ranges

Exercises ⟶ 1 to 4 & 8   8   5 to 9

	10	1000
	5	500
	1	100
	0.5	50
	.4	
	.3	
	.2	
	0.1	10
	0.05	5
	0.01	1

10   20   Time   30   40   50

Suggested ranges

Exercises ⟶ 1 to 4 & 8   5 to 9

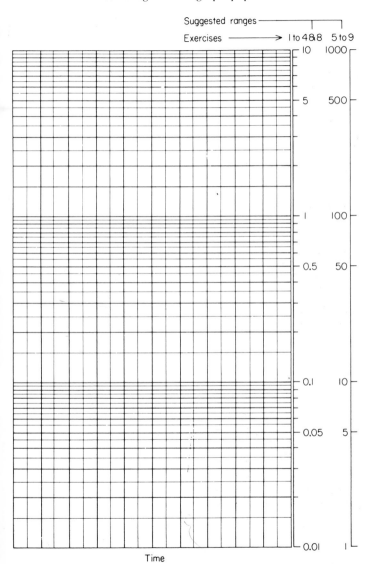

Time

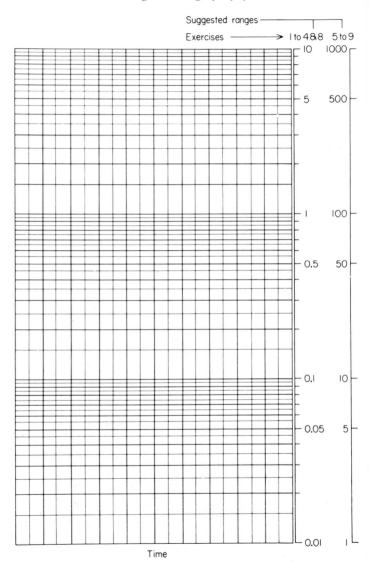

Time

Suggested ranges

Exercises ———→ 1 to 4&8 5 to 9

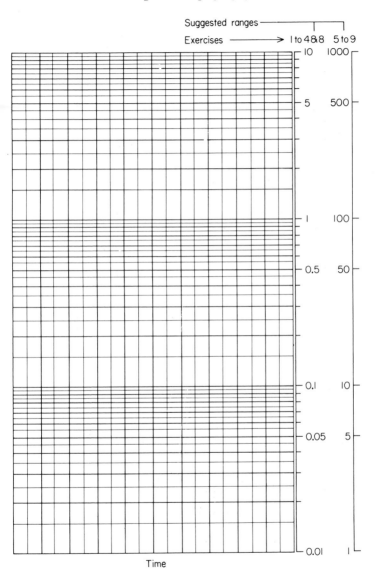

Time

108   *Semi-logarithmic graph paper*

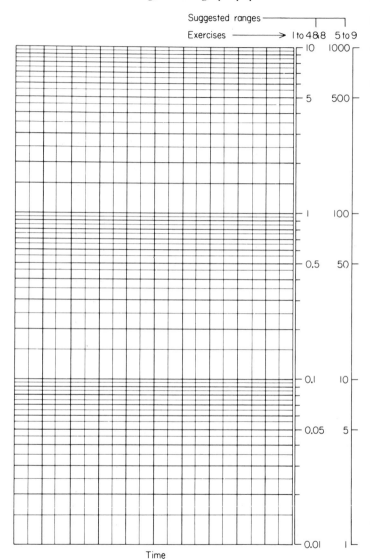

Suggested ranges

Exercises ⟶ 1 to 4 & 8   5 to 9

Time

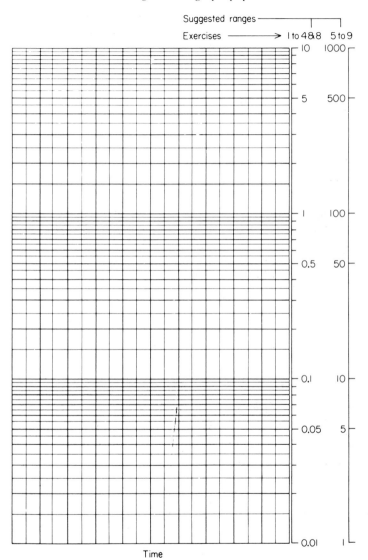

Suggested ranges

Exercises ⟶ 1 to 4 & 8   5 to 9

Time

Semi-logarithmic graph paper

Suggested ranges
Exercises ⟶ 1 to 4 & 8 5 to 9

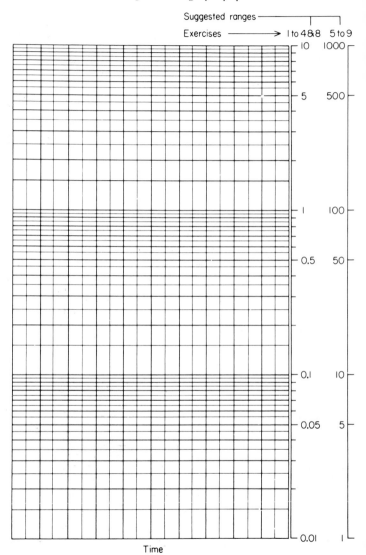

Time

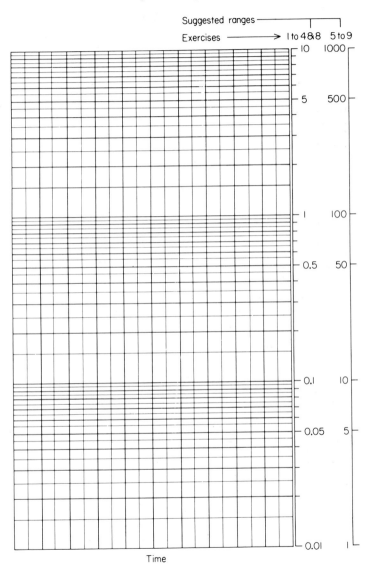

Suggested ranges

Exercises ⟶ 1 to 4&8   5 to 9

Time

Suggested ranges

Exercises ⟶ 1 to 4 & 8   5 to 9

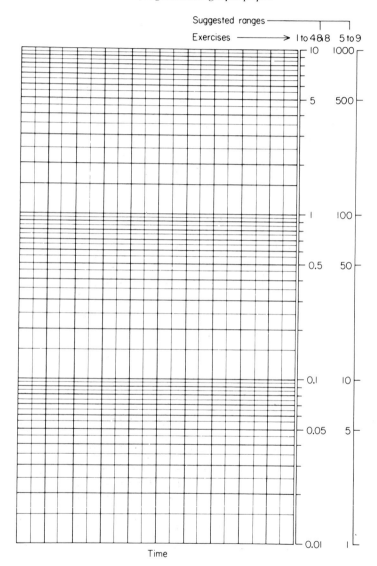

Time

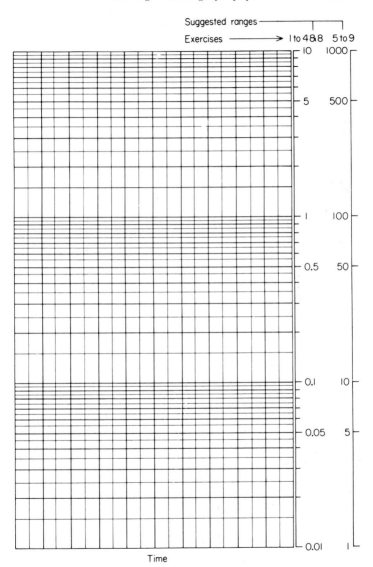

Time

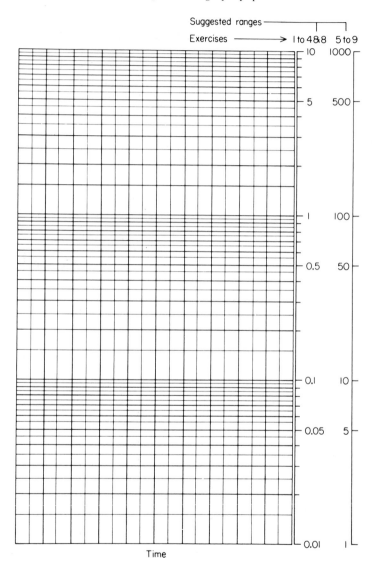

Suggested ranges

Exercises ⟶ 1 to 4 & 8   5 to 9

Time

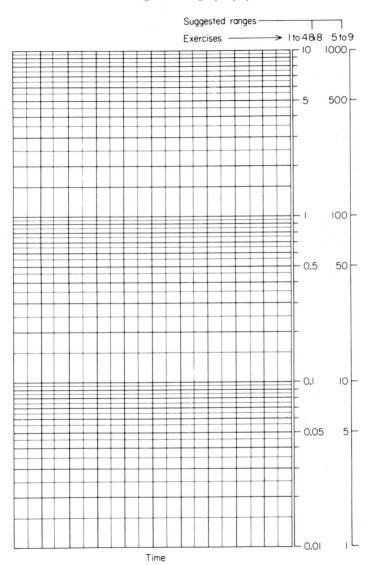

Suggested ranges

Exercises ⟶ 1 to 4 & 8   5 to 9

Time

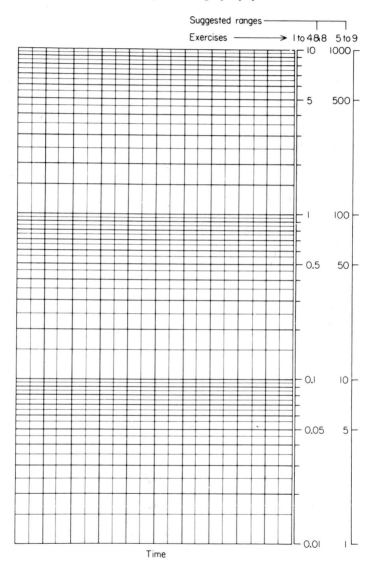

Suggested ranges

Exercises ⟶ 1 to 4 & 8 5 to 9

Time

Index